ESSENTIAL OILS

FOR BEGINNERS

THE EASY GUIDEBOOK TO GET STARTED WITH ESSENTIAL OILS AND AROMATHERAPY

Author

Amanda Robinson

CONTENT

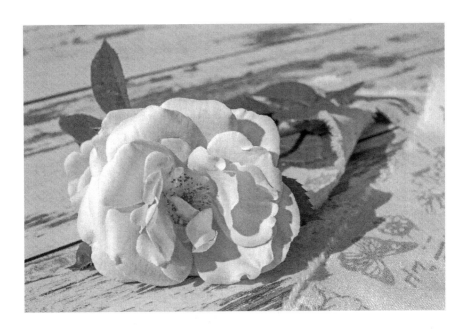

INTRODUCTION

Have you ever wondered relieving the headache that is bugging you since morning without eating Ibuprofen?

Do you know how to calm your allergies without anti-analgesics?

Did you ever achieve success in healing your burn without rushing to the skin specialist?

Or have you ever wondered about normalizing your raised blood pressure or turning the switch of your watery nose off without some sort of medication?

Are you suffering from Anxiety, Depression, Stress?

Feeling tired or aching?

Do you want to calm it all down anytime soon?

Searching for relief?

∗∗∗

If this has ever been what you are looking for, you are at the right place. We have got the answers for all of this.

Essential oils and Aromatherapy is all that you need. They are not only beneficial in the above-mentioned conditions. There are a lot of benefits of Essential oils and Aromatherapy, both health-related and other everyday use benefits.

Now, when you have got the answer, you need to start getting to know about the marvels of Essential oils and the benefits you can achieve from Aromatherapy.

We have got it all covered.
Here, you will get to know about how the essential oils are formed, their source and extraction methods. A brief introduction and history to everything are always welcomed, right. You will also learn about the compounds that have therapeutic benefits close to essential oils and are used in aromatherapy.

The knowledge of Aromatherapy is as important as that of the Essential oils. While learning about the types of benefits you can obtain from the Aromatherapy, you will also learn How to obtain them.
The choice of essential oil marks the beginning of Aromatherapy.
The use of the right carrier oil for the respective essential oil along with the correct technique will not only minimize the

fear of allergic reaction (if any) but will also help in maximizing the benefits of this holistic therapeutic treatment.

Excited to learn more about it?

Let's get started!

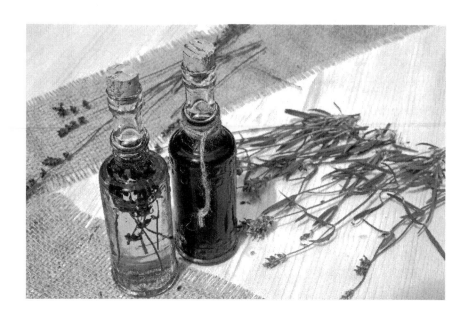

CHAPTER 1

INTRODUCTION TO ESSENTIAL OILS

Before moving on to an explained introduction, history, benefits and choice of an Essential oil, let's first have a look at the list below. This includes a pre-reading guide to what you will learn in this first chapter of the book on Essential oils and Aromatherapy.

What is an Essential oil?

> Definition
> Source
> Meaning of the word 'Essential
> Meaning of the word 'Oil
> Extraction Method
> Administration Method
> Other names given to Essential oils

A Brief History of Essential oils

> The Aristotelian Idea
> Evolution of the Term, 'Essential Oils'
> Identification of Therapeutic Benefits
> Discovery of Anti-Viral Benefits

Benefits of Essential oils

> Health Benefits
> Other Benefits

How to make the Right Choice of an Essential oil?

> Difference between Essential oil and Fragrance oil

In the pages to come, each of these mentioned above will be covered in detail for a better understanding of Essential oils.

Let's brainstorm. Have you ever experienced the rose scent? If yes, you have enjoyed the aromatic benefit of an essential oil. The scent of rose is because of the essential oil of the rose plant.

Definition

Essential oil, as the name suggests, is an important extract that is infused with quality compounds to provide benefits to its user. They are strongly fragranced liquids that are not friends with water, that is, they do not dissolve in water like fresh juice does. Moreover, if they are left uncovered, they will evaporate in the air making the whole surrounding fragranced.

Remember something from high school chemistry? Volatile, aromatic, hydrophobic? These three words are the definition of essential oils. They have been explained in the above paragraph as well. Considering the qualities of essential oils, the definition of Essential oils will be,

"An Essential oil is a concentrated hydrophobic, volatile aromatic extract of plants in nature."

Source

As the essential oils are plant extracts in nature, the source of essential oils becomes the herbaceous and beneficial plants. They are extracted from all parts of a plant including its stem, leaves, flowers, bark, seeds, roots and any other living part of the plant. These parts are chosen because of the abundance of aromatic compounds in them.

Meaning of the word 'Essential.'

We are familiar with the word essential as 'of extreme importance.' The same annotation was used for essential amino acids because of their extreme importance in normal body functioning. However, the word 'Essential' here is not an imitation from the word essential amino acids. The word essential is given to them because they are responsible for imparting the plant its fragrance. In simple words, they make a rose, a Rose because of its characteristic essence.

Meaning of the word 'Oil.'

What comes to your mind when you hear or read the word, oil? Coconut oil, with oily touch, right? The word 'Oil' in the Essential oil is not because it is an oil. It does not provide an oily feeling upon touch. It is a misnomer which means that being an extract, it is given the name oil. It has no such fatty acid properties. If any essential oil contains an oily touch, it is impure and has been diluted by any other pure oil.

Extraction Method

The essential oils are extracted from various plant parts by a process known as steam distillation or water distillation. In this process, the essential compound or concentrates (hydrophobic, volatile aromatic) are converted into steam in the first step. The evaporated compounds are collected and then converted back into a concentrated liquid form. The product obtained is a pure Essential oil containing all the beneficial properties and aroma.

Administration Method

Even though the guideline of administration of Essential oils will be provided in detail in Chapter No. 3, the basic information will be provided here. The three methods used commonly for the application and administration of essential oils include

i.   the direct ingestion of essential oils
ii. the diffusion of essential oils followed by inhalation
iii. the topical application of essential oils

The **ingestion** of an essential oil can be done as per required. The methods used are suppositories and the oral ingestion of essential oil. However, for the oral ingestion, the presence of a certified health care provider is mandatory.

The benefits of essential oils can be obtained by **inhaling** them. The methods advised are the use of a diffuser, dry evaporation using cotton balls, steam inhalation, and as aerosol sprays. However, the steam inhalation is not recommended under 7 years of age. The older individuals are advised to wear swimming goggles to protect their eyes.

For the **topical** application, the methods used are massaging, baths, compresses and sprays. Moreover, the essential oils can be irritating to the skin when concentrated. It is usually advised to dilute them prior application.

These three methods can be exploited in various ways which will be discussed later. Their usage depends on the type of benefit required of them.

Other names given to Essential oils

Just so you know, the other names given to essential oil are oils of the 'plant name' (from which they are extracted), ethereal oils, volatile oils and atherolea oils respectively. Keep that in mind while on a hunt for them.

The Aristotelian Idea

The history of Essential oils starts from the Aristotelian idea about the matter. According to him, the matter is composed primarily of four elements namely of water, fire, earth, and air. Soon after gaining popularity, the idea of the presence of another element in the matter, the fifth one, which is called quintessence emerged. The quintessence is composed of spirit force.

Evolution of the Term, 'Essential Oils'

More than thousand years ago, the philosophers and researchers believed that the removal of the spirits from the plants results in a powerful potion. It was believed that this potion would provide all the therapeutic, medicinal and spiritual benefits to its users. This potion can be extracted by the process of evaporation and distillation. It was made possible in the 11th Century after the discovery of steam distillation. So, an extraction of the "quintessential oils" lead to the term "Essential Oils" in the ancient times.

Identification of Therapeutic Benefits

With the passage of time, the researchers identified the compounds responsible for providing a plant with its immune system. The compounds responsible were the same that can be extracted in the form of essential oils. This discovery provided the basis to the concept that the same compounds responsible for the plant immune system and protection can also provide protection and immunity to its users.

In the years to come, it was proved that the essential oils could not only help in boosting immunity but is also responsible for providing other medicinal and therapeutic benefit. The benefits will be discussed later in detail. However, one extremely important discovery over this concept till date is the use of essential oils as anti-viral agents.

Wait, What?

Buckle up. Essential oils can be used as an anti-viral agent. Need Proof? Here we have it.

Continue Reading!

Discovery of Anti-Viral Benefits

Till now, we all are well familiar with the infectious property of viruses. We have also realized that antibiotics have no control over them. This is because the viruses have the property of replicating within living cells and antibiotics lacked the property of penetrating a living cell. Thus, they do not provide any useful effect when it comes to treating viruses. So, we have received an open **Sorry** from Antibiotics!

However, a recent study conducted by Wu Shuhua, Patel Krupa B and colleagues in 2010 provided scientific evidence to the World community that essential oils have the property of penetrating the living cells. You heard it right. Not only penetrating but significantly attenuating viral activity and thus killing the viruses. Isn't it too good to be true?

This extremely beneficial property and its scientific evidence were provided by a study on influenza virus infection. It was an in vitro study which was conducted on the MDCK cells (Wu. S et al., 2010). This lead to the discovery of essential oils as an antiviral agent providing a new direction and **Hope** to the scientific and therapeutic community. This has not only opened new ways towards research but has also increased the motivation in the scientific community towards fighting the Viruses.

We understand that you are here for understanding the health benefits of Essential oils. But we have additional perks here as well. Stay tuned!

There are more than a hundred uses of these essential oils. If we divide them based on the purposes they are used, they are extremely helpful in healthcare, cleaning and as a home accessory. Yes, other than healthcare.

Health Benefits

An essential oil is the most powerful and effective source of well-being when it comes to addressing a range of physical, spiritual and emotional Conditions. Essential oils provide these benefits without the threat of lethal and fatal side effects. The side effects which are commonly associated with allopathic pharmaceuticals.

The essential oils have anti-microbial properties by nature which determines that most of them are either antibacterial or have properties like those of antifungal materials. They are also blessed with anti-parasitic properties and antiviral properties. This provides them with the benefits of antibacterial, antifungal and that of an antiviral agent

The essential oils are also used as natural remedies and medicines for relieving several complications. Healing burns, relieving migraines, sinusitis, bronchitis, eczema, and psoriasis, reducing fever, curbing food cravings, motion sickness, healing blisters and relieving sunburn to name a few.

Other Benefits

There are a lot of uses of these essential oils besides in the health industry. They are very beneficial for skin and are used in the spa treatments, relaxations, skin care and end for enhancing beauty. They can also be used to make the homemade products such as chocolate peppermint ice cream, homemade toothpaste, homemade soap, homemade deodorant and eczema creams. They are also used in making the homemade cleansing wipes, baby wipes, home cleaners, hand sanitizers and lip balms.

These benefits not only restrict essential oils to the health industry, rather they are extremely diverse in nature and effects. They encourage utilization of essential oils in the skincare, cleaning and homemade products to acquire maximum benefits.

How to make the Right Choice of an Essential oil?

Now that you have acquired the important introductory information about the essential oils, it is the time to understand how crucial it is to choose the **Right** essential oil. This does not mean that you have acquired every information needed, as the rest of the chapters cover the understanding to everything about essential oils and aromatherapy. This topic will, however, tell you what should be kept in mind along with opening your eyes to something branded similar to an essential oil. Let's continue!

The choice of essential oils is completely dependent on the purpose it is being used for. And that will determine which one is suitable to be used and when? Is it being used for treating allergies, inflammations, burns, fungal infections or the purpose is to relax and stabilize the mood? A mature choice will help in acquiring benefits from an essential oil.

Before applying or using an essential oil, it is highly advised to consult a specialist and perform an extensive research. The essential oils are 80 to 100 times more concentrated then they are in plants. Researching about the benefits and side effects will help in making a mature choice. This will ensure the gain of maximum benefits while minimizing the experience of any harmful effects.

Difference between Essential oil and Fragrance oil

Essential oils are certified and 100% pure organic compound, extracted solely from plant source by steam distillation without the addition of any chemical. Thus, the important consideration here which must be kept in mind is that for the application and administration, the essential oils used must be certified 100% authentic.

There is a type of aromatic oils called the fragrance oil which is similar in fragrance and appearance to the essential oil. The main difference here is that the fragrance oil is artificial, produced synthetically and composed of chemicals. They are not fit for consumption and have no therapeutic benefits. They are categorized under the umbrella of essential oils in some places, or the slight alteration in labeling can be misleading.

One must be watchful in this aspect to avoid the application of a similar 80 to 100 times concentrated fragrance oil, herbicide, pesticide, chemical fertilizer or an insecticide to your body or to the body of someone you care about a lot. This will prevent the incidents of harmful allergies, infections and side effects.

Keeping in Mind

- Essential oils are certified and 100% pure organic compound, extracted solely from plant source by steam distillation without the addition of any chemical.
- For getting benefits, essential oils can be inhaled, ingested or applied topically.
- Essential oils provide the benefits of antibacterial, antifungal and antiviral agent.
- Only certified and 100% pure, Essential oils, must be the choice of use.

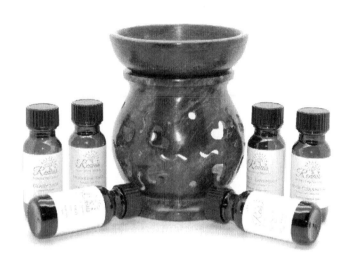

CHAPTER 2

INTRODUCTION TO AROMATHERAPY

You just completed your First Chapter. Now, you have a good knowledge of Essential oils. Good Work!

Excited about getting to know Aromatherapy? We are more eager to share the information. But before moving on, let's first have a look at the list below. A pre-reading guide is always Welcome, isn't it? This list will tell you what you will learn in the second chapter of the book on starter guide to Essential oils and Aromatherapy.

What is an Aromatherapy?

Definition
When is Aromatherapy Used?
How to Perform an Aromatherapy
Purpose of the Aromatherapy

Brief History of Aromatherapy

The term Aromatherapy
Theory behind the Practice of Aromatherapy

Compounds used in Aromatherapy

Aromatherapy Oils
Additional oils

Benefits of Aromatherapy

Health Benefits
Spiritual Benefits

Is Aromatherapy the Right Choice?

Is it Safe or Unsafe?

In the pages to come, each of these mentioned above will be covered in detail for a better understanding of Essential oils.

What is an Aromatherapy?

Ever been to a spa? Or Some pretty aroma that took you in, totally? Soothing and Calming? You have been near to the experience of Aromatherapy.

Definition

Aromatherapy is the use of natural oils to achieve benefits. The use of this therapy is known to provide psychological and physical wellbeing. In this therapy, the aroma-producing oils and extracts that are plants in nature are used to treat allergies and illnesses. It is widely believed that the inhalation of aromatic compounds positively stimulates the functions of the brain.

When is Aromatherapy Used?

Aromatherapy is often offered as a complementary treatment or in the form of an alternative therapy. Now, you would be wondering what a complementary treatment is? What does an alternative therapy mean? Hold on; it will be explained in a second.

i. **Complementary Treatment:**

Complementary treatment is usually offered along with the conventional treatment of a disease.

ii. **Alternative Therapy:**

Alternative therapy is offered as a new treatment instead of the conventional treatment for a certain disease.

An aromatherapy can be used alone as an alternative treatment or along with the conventional treatment as a complementary therapy. **Bonus**, Right?

How to Perform an Aromatherapy?

To perform aromatherapy, the services of Aromatherapists are utilized. They are the specialists of performing aromatherapy. In the first step, a blend of pure organic aromatic compounds or an essential oil with some other substance like a carrier oil, a lotion or alcohol is prepared. The blend can then be utilized in different ways.

The aromatherapy blend can either be dispersed in the air and inhaled. The blend can be sprayed or applied directly to the skin to let it get absorbed. It can be poured into water to have a good water bath. The aromatherapy blend can also be massaged into the skin, however, for direct application onto the skin; there are certain cautions to be kept in mind. These will be discussed in later chapters.

These methods are for obtaining maximum benefits out of aromatherapy and depend solely on the preference and the type of treatment required.

Purpose of the Aromatherapy

Coming to the purpose of the aromatherapy, it is to relieve muscle stress, fight illness and cure a variety of medical conditions. It is used to initiate the muscle relaxation which is done in a way to release the stress off, of them. A similar study has shown that fragrance produced by certain essential oils stimulates the production of substances that are involved in relieving and fighting pain in the body.

The aromatherapy is also involved in curbing a variety of medical conditions that are both physical and mental. These conditions include the following

   i.   Burns,
   ii. Depression,
   iii. Infection,
   iv. Insomnia and
   v.   High Blood Pressure

The use of aromatherapy in the above mention conditions help in accelerating the treatment process, if not curing.

History is the best part of any study. It reminds one of the importance by bringing forth the efforts put into it while researching. To honor those who worked for our today, let's just get a brief knowledge of Aromatherapy history before moving on to the benefits.

The term Aromatherapy

The aromatherapy originated in Europe to cure minor illnesses, and this therapy is in practice since the start of the 20th Century. In 1907, a relatively small number of doctors and scientists incorporated aromatherapy into their clinical and research practice. However, the term 'Aromatherapy' was first coined in the book by René Maurice Gatte Fossé, a French Chemist in 1937. The book was named "Aromathérapie: Les Huiles Essentielles, Hormones Végétales."

For research purpose, Gatte Fossé badly burnt his hand and then treated it with the lavender oil using Aromatherapy, to prove his point. This is mentioned in his book as well. This provided the world a new direction in research. During World War II, the medicinal benefits of Aromatherapy were introduced to the World by Jean Valnet, a French surgeon. With the publication of his findings, the aromatherapy was widely exploited by the medical and therapeutic industry in the mid of 20th Century.

In 1993, English adaptation of Gatte Fossé's book was published. After the publication of English adaptation, the advancement in therapeutic domain took an irreversible turn, for good. Today, we are using Aromatherapy to curb allergies and infection. We have incorporated this therapy with other treatments to obtain maximum benefits, which is why the nowaday's use of aromatherapy as a spiritual treatment is gaining the most popularity.

No jokes, Aromatherapy and Essential oils have changed our lives, in a good way.

Theory behind the Practice of Aromatherapy

The practitioners and the specialists believe that the fragrances of plants are extracted in the form of an essential oil. The essential oil aroma stimulates the nerves present in the nose. These stimulated nerves and impulses are responsible for sending the signal to the part of the brain that controls emotions and memory. This belief is the theory behind the practice of aromatherapy.

The result of the aromatherapy can be either calming the nerves or stimulating them depending on the type of oil used and the kind of effect required.

Compounds used in Aromatherapy

There are several compounds used in the aromatherapy. Most of them and not all of them are purely plant extracts. There are two types of compounds used in aromatherapy. One is Aromatherapy oils, and the other is Additional oils.

Aromatherapy Oils

They are the fundamental compounds used in the aromatherapy. Aromatherapy oils are mainly composed of the following

i.   Essential Oils
ii.   extracted concentrated Absolutes
iii.   Carbon Dioxide CO_2 Extracts
iv.   Hydrosols
v.   and Carrier Oils

These compounds utilized commonly in the aromatherapy differ in their methods of extraction, distillation, their aromatic composition, and purity. The general curtain used to refer to these all, and the naturally occurring volatile aromatic compounds and oils from plants, absolutes, and carbon dioxide, etc. is the Aromatherapy Oils.

An important consideration here is that among all, only the Essential oils are 100% organic which means they are only the plant volatile aromatic extract. This condition is essential for labeling an oil an essential oil as it is their distinguishing feature. The absolutes, carbon dioxide extracts, hydrosols are often curtained under Essential oil; they are not. Moreover, one must be watchful of the fragrance oils often mislead as an essential oil. They are not either.

Additional oils

Along with the above-mentioned compounds, the aromatherapy is also found encouraging the use of some other complementary ingredients that are present in nature. They are:

i. Jojoba (liquid wax)
ii. Vegetable oils (cold pressed)
iii. Milk Powders
iv. Herbs
v. Clays
vi. Sugar (as an exfoliant)
vii. Sea Salts
viii. Muds

These ingredients are responsible for mediating the process of aromatherapy by acting as a carrier or a facilitator.

There are several benefits of Aromatherapy. The only way to obtain the countless benefits of the aromatherapy to its maximum requires a good insight of the aromatherapy, essential oils and the usage methods. The purpose of using them in an aromatherapy and the purpose of aromatherapy must be very clear. In addition to that, a good know-how of other materials used in the aromatherapy will only result in helping and aiding in achieving benefits.

Now, that you have read the instructions, the time has come to know some basic benefits you can achieve from aromatherapy. A number health and spiritual benefits will be explained below.

Health Benefits

To name a few, given below is the list of highly important health benefits that you can obtain with the use of aromatherapy.

i. It can relieve stress
ii. Aromatherapy has the capacity of acting as an antidepressant
iii. Aromatherapy helps in reviving memory
iv. Energy levels can be boosted by aromatherapy
v. It aids in the process of healing and in recovery
vi. It helps in relieving headaches
vii. Aromatherapy helps in balancing sleep cycle
viii. It aids the body's immune system
ix. Aromatherapy can relieve pain

x.   It improves the digestive system

These health benefits if exploited fully can result in a quality health and lifestyle of an individual.

Spiritual Benefits

Aromatherapy, according to the spiritual experts is a very good source of obtaining peace. A few of the spiritual benefits are mentioned below.

   i.   Aid in sleep
  ii.   Promoting peaceful sleep
 iii.   A sense of protection
  iv.   Spiritual connection with the Prophets
   v.   A sense of oneness with Earth
  vi.   A feeling of purification of body
 vii.   An increase in inner vision
viii.   Stimulation of a conscious mind
  ix.   Bring the heart to peace
   x.   Allow the heart to trust
  xi.   Inner enlightenment

One thing should be kept in mind for the spiritual benefits that they are known to provide peace to spirits, and there is no scientific evidence to prove them.

This does not mark an end to the benefits of Aromatherapy. Keep Reading; the book is filled with them.

Is Aromatherapy the Right Choice?

Like every other person, you will be worried as to why are you reading this? Does it do what it says? Do you really need this information? We can understand. While conducting the research, we came across this thought a dozen times. I will explain it, Right choice or not? You will decide it very soon.

Clinical Aromatherapist Cary Caster who not only spent her 20 years studying essential oils around the World but is also the Founder of 21 Drops. In her words, people, especially practitioners underestimate the power of nose and sense of smell. It is the most primitive sense that has an immediate effect on the brain.

What do you want to achieve when you are exposed to headaches? **Think!**

What an ibuprofen or a painkiller does in this case scenario? **Recall!**

The only exposure a common person would have with Aromatherapy is while having a spa treatment. But do you remember the after effects? Relaxation, beautiful skin and freshness!

Exactly these steps are played during treatment. The drugs involved in relieving the pain only reduce the sensation of pain by masking it for a few hours. But this is not the actual remedy. Is it? The actual treatment would be the eradication of pain by effecting on the causes.

The headache is usually caused by the stress and

Aromatherapy works in steps to get rid of it.

i. it relieves the stress,
ii. ease the pain and
iii. refresh the blood.
iv. induce immunity

All of this is achieved by bringing the fresh blood to the brain. Isn't it the ultimate remedy?

Exactly this happens in almost all the Aromatherapy procedures. The condition might differ, the choice of essential oil will change, a different carrier oil can be used. But the result will be phenomenal.

Doesn't it make the Aromatherapy, the **Right Choice?**

Is it Safe or Unsafe?

Aromatherapy has always been caught up in the plight of Safe or Unsafe. While everybody seems to be really concerned when it comes to safety in Aromatherapy, the safety in every other medical procedure is set behind. This is not a justification; however, it must be kept in mind that the side effects of any treatment can be potential when it comes to artificial treatment.

In the case of natural treatment, like in Aromatherapy, there are benefits only. Everything is good until the right procedures are followed. There are a few bad effects that can arise only if the procedural instructions and safety guides are not followed. They will be discussed in later chapters.

With every good, there comes a bad in handy; the rule that applies everywhere. It is when things are not taken care of or when the precautions and instruction are taken for granted. A few of the considerations are mentioned below. However, a detailed guide to methodology and precautions with all Do's and Don'ts will be explained in detail in the coming chapters.

Dilution of Essential oil

The essential oils used in aromatherapy can pose a serious threat if not diluted, as they need dilution in most cases prior use, with a carrier oil or an added lotion.

Avoid Direct Application and Ingestion

Being highly concentrated, they can cause irritation upon inhalation, infection or inflammation upon their direct application onto the skin and serious damage if ingested orally.

Addition of Carrier oil

The addition of some carrier oil in the essential oil is recommended for the aromatherapy purposes. The carrier oil maybe olive oil, jojoba oil or coconut oil among others.

Aromatherapy is not recommended without the addition of carrier oil in the essential oils. The details of how the aromatherapy can be conducted with the added carrier oils in the essential oils will be covered in Chapter No. 7, Aromatic compositions.

Keeping in Mind

- Aromatherapy is the use of natural oils to achieve psychological and physical wellbeing.
- It can be used as a complementary or an alternative treatment.
- It is performed by making a blend of essential oil and a carrier oil.
- Aromatherapy is used to achieve various benefits.
- There are two types of compounds used in Aromatherapy; Aromatherapy oils and Additional oils.
- Aromatherapy is capable of providing numerous health and spiritual benefits.
- Aromatherapy seems to be the right choice of treatment considering the type of beneficial effects it produces.
- The safety of an Aromatherapy procedure depends upon various factors.3
- Abiding by the procedural details and precautionary measures is the only way to achieve maximum benefits from Aromatherapy

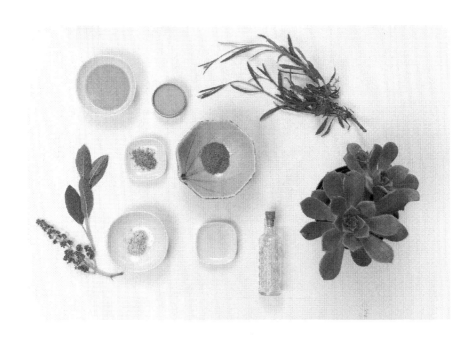

CHAPTER 3

TYPOLOGY OF AROMATHERAPY OILS

AND OTHER AROMATIC INGREDIENTS

The first two Chapters that you just completed were a detailed introduction to Essential oils and Aromatherapy. We know that Aromatherapy is used as a complementary or alternative treatment requires the use of pure and organic ingredients. The purity and originality are given a lot of importance and stress when it comes to performing the aromatherapy. That is why, only natural and pure carrier oils, essential oils, resins, etc. are used in the aromatherapy.

Now that you are well familiar with the two very important

terminologies, it is time to move onto the next step. Excited?

In the first chapter of the second phase of learning, we will learn about all the oils and ingredients that are used in an Aromatherapy. They are Aromatherapy oils and other Aromatic ingredients.

But wait, why not we list the content of the third chapter before starting it? Below is a pre-reading guide to what you will learn in the third chapter of the book about Essential oils and Aromatherapy.

Aromatherapy Oils

- Absolutes

   Difference between Essential oils and Absolutes
   Nature of Chemical Solvent used in the extraction of Absolutes
   The Fate of the Chemical Solvent used in Absolutes Extraction
   Amount of Chemical Solvent Present in Absolutes after Purification
   Absolutes; a preference in Aromatherapy or Not?
   Why a Different Method?
   What is in Absolutes which is not in Essential oils?
   The Use of Absolutes, Is it Safe?

- Carbon dioxide Extracts

   Extraction Method of Carbon Dioxide Extracts
   Difference between Absolutes and Carbon Dioxide Extracts
   The advantage over Essential oils?

Fragrance Oil

Floral Essences

Following the list, we know, there will be a hundred questions that bombarded you. But why stuff your mind right up here, when you are going to learn about them all in the coming pages while reading.

Hold on!

- The list above will be explained in detail where almost all the questions relating to them will be answered.

As explained in the second chapter, aromatherapy oils are the oils, ingredients that are obtained from the therapeutic plant source and are used in the practice of holistic aromatherapy. They are same as all of them are extracted from a plant source. They are different in terms of their extraction method and the purity of plant content extracted. **Makes sense?**

It will! The aromatherapy oils, are

- Essential oils
- Absolutes
- Carbon dioxide Extracts
- Carrier Oils
- Infused Oils or Macerated Oils

They are all discussed in details below apart from Essential oils as they are Explained in Chapter No. 1 in detail of this book.

Grab some popcorns!

Essential oils

Essential oils are the pure plant extracts used in the holistic aromatherapy. They are 100% organic extracted from a plant by steam distillation. They have the strong aroma of the plant they are extracted from and are known as hydrophobic, aromatic plant extracts with a volatile nature.

For more understanding, scroll back to Chapter No. 1. *Introduction to Essential oils.* Moreover, they will be covered in the coming chapters as well.

Absolutes

The second used aromatherapy oil is Absolutes. They are extracted from plants and are highly aromatic in their composition. Absolutes are extracted in the form of liquid.

Isn't is all exactly like their counterparts called Essential oils? (explained in Chapter No. 1).

Absolutes are closest to the essential oils in composition and properties. So, what makes them different? Let's find out.

Difference between Essential oils and Absolutes

The only difference that sketches a line between essential oils and absolutes is their method of extraction. The essential oils as explained earlier are extracted by either water or steam distillation. While in the extraction of absolutes, some sort of solvents that are chemical in nature are used.

The use of a chemical solvent in absolute extraction is the only thing that makes the two stand apart.

Nature of Chemical Solvent used in the extraction of Absolutes

The chemical solvent usually used in the extraction of absolutes is hexane. It is an alkaline solvent with the chemical formula C_6H_{14}. This six-carbon compound is citrus in nature and is an extraction solvent. It is used to extract solvents in food production. A small fraction of volatile hexane is also present in guava, apple, orange and heated sweet potatoes.

The Fate of the Chemical Solvent used in Absolutes Extraction

The chemical solvent used in absolutes extraction is removed in the final stage. However, when the absolutes were observed after purification, a scanty amount of that chemical solvent was still left behind in the absolute. This confirms that even after the removal of the chemical in the final stage of the absolute production, a small amount of it is present in the final aromatic extracted product.

Amount of Chemical Solvent Present in Absolutes after Purification

Aromatic absolutes are extracted with extreme care and precision to ensure maximum removal of the chemical solvent. Even with this precision, a small amount is present in the final product. It has been confirmed that the chemical solvent in the absolutes is extremely scarce and almost negligible. Moreover, it is not found affecting the aromatic properties of the absolutes in any way.

Absolutes; a preference in Aromatherapy or Not?

Within the holistic aromatherapy scope, the steam or water distilled essentials oils are given preference over solvent extracted aromatic absolutes.

It is not said that absolutes are totally left aside, as they are used in some of the holistic aromatherapy practices. The thing is that they are not the first preference in the aromatherapy practice, it is essential oils. Moreover, if both the absolutes and essential oils are present for the same purpose, the essential oil is given preference over aromatic absolutes.

Now that the difference between Essential oils and Absolutes is clear, a solid question knocks the door.

The Method of Extraction of the Aromatic Oil used for some Plants is by Solvent as in the case of Absolutes rather than by Steam or Water Distillation as in the case of Essential Oils.

Why a Different Method?

The answer to this question requires some brainstorming. There must be some valid reason for skipping steam distillation and opting solvent. Right?

The case when steam distillation is used to extract the natural aromatic ingredients of precious plants. The resultant is in the form of essential oils. There are two issues in this case,

i. Either the resultant has less natural oil or concentrate (in the quality or quantity)

ii. or the plant does not withstand the steam distillation treatment and get harmed.

In either of these cases, the other method used to extract a quality and quantity natural aromatic concentrate, is by utilizing the chemical solvent extraction method.

What is in Absolutes which is not in Essential oils?

Well, the method utilized is chemical solvent extraction and steam distillation. There must be some bargain? Shouldn't there be?

So, there is!

The concentrate obtained as the result of chemical solvent extraction is a lot more concentrated than the extract or concentrate obtained as the result of steam distillation. More concentrated than 80%. **WOW!**

It is famous about the essential oils that they are rich in natural aromatic content and are highly concentrated. However, the aromatic absolutes are far more concentrated and rich in the aromatic content than essential oils.

The use of Absolutes, is it Safe?

It is extremely important to know that even though the aromatic absolutes are used in the holistic aromatherapy, they must be used with great precision and care. Whether the concentration of solvent is scanty and negligible, it must be utilized with caution.

In addition to it, some of the essential oils can be of great benefit when taken internally. The recommendation source should always be practitioners and experts for the internal administration of essential oils. However, the absolutes are never recommended for any sort of internal administration and application.

So, the Absolutes contain more aromatic content and are highly concentrated, even more than the Essential oils. But this presence of a chemical solvent, though negligible, makes them a Second Choice!

Carbon dioxide Extracts

The most used component in aromatherapy besides Essential oils is Carbon Dioxide Extracts. The oils or concentrates extracted by using the carbon dioxide method from plants are called Carbon Dioxide Extracts. The other names assigned to them are the carbon dioxide supercritical extract or simply the carbon dioxides in the field of aromatherapy.

Extraction Method of Carbon Dioxide Extracts

The extraction of the carbon dioxide extracts is done by using the method called supercritical carbon dioxide method of extraction.

Supercritical Carbon Dioxide Extraction Method?

Such a Critical Name. Let's repeat. Super-Critical Carbon Dioxide Extraction Method. Seems fine now!

As the name suggests, it is Super Critical.

In the supercritical carbon dioxide extraction method, liquefied carbon dioxide is used and not the gaseous one present in the atmosphere. The atmospheric carbon dioxide is collected and pressurized. The pressure converts it into its liquid form. The liquefied carbon dioxide is thus used as the solvent here like a chemical solvent used in the extraction of the absolutes.

The natural aromatic components present in the plant are extracted in the liquid carbon dioxide. After collection, the recovery of the carbon dioxide extracts is done by releasing the pressure from liquefied carbon dioxide. The release of pressure changes the form of carbon from liquid to gas. The gaseous carbon is then released into the air, leaving behind the carbon dioxide extracts only.

Done! The Carbon Dioxide Extracts are in hand.

I was not that Critical anyway!

Difference between Absolutes and Carbon Dioxide Extracts

Unlike absolutes, the carbon dioxide extracts are not obtained and extracted using a chemical solvent. Thus, carbon dioxide extracts do not have any chemical remains in them. The atmospheric carbon dioxide is pressurized to liquid and is used in the liquid form. The pressure is released later which releases the gas into the atmosphere. Back to where it belonged. The departure of gas leaves the pure extract behind, that is, carbon dioxide extract.

No Chemical, No Impurity.

Advantage over Essential oils?

The carbon dioxide extraction has an advantage over the steam distilled essential oil extraction. The former does not pose any sort of threat to plant in respect to damage caused by heat.

Too Good, Right?

Types of Carbon Dioxide Extracts

The carbon dioxide extracts are now increasingly finding their way in the market because of their advantages. There are two types of carbon dioxide supercritical extracts available. They are.

Carbon Dioxide Selects

Carbon Dioxide Totals

These two types are explained below in detail.

Carbon Dioxide Selects:

Carbon dioxide selects are created by using <u>low-pressure method</u> to convert carbon dioxide into liquid. The carbon dioxide selects generally contains the volatile aromatic components of the plants that are soluble in the solvent, liquid carbon dioxide. There are different aromatic molecules that are present in a plant. Some are lighter while some are heavier. The heavier ones are unable to be distilled by the steam distillation method. Thus, comes in the carbon dioxide selects that have solubilized the heavier aromatic molecules. That is why the carbon dioxide selects smell more like the natural herbs than the essential oils extracted by steam distillation.

Carbon Dioxide Totals:

The carbon dioxide totals are created by <u>exerting heavy pressure</u> to liquefy carbon dioxide. The carbon dioxide totals contain almost all the molecules that are soluble in liquid carbon dioxide. That is why the carbon dioxide totals are much heavier than the carbon dioxide selects. They not only contain the heavier volatile aromatic carbon dioxide soluble molecules in them but also the liquid carbon dioxide soluble waxes, natural lipids, and other related molecules present in the plants.

So, Carbon Dioxide Extracts are Pure and Do not harm the plant unlike Absolutes and Essential oils respectively. They are the Future!

Carrier Oils

Let's just cut short, long paragraphs and understand Carrier oils in the easiest way possible.

"Derived from the fatty portion of a botanical, a carrier oil is, in fact, a vegetable oil that is being extracted from the kernels, seeds and the nuts."

Advantage over Essential oils, Absolutes and Carbon dioxide extracts

Unlike essential oils, carbon dioxide extracts and absolutes, that cause severe irritation, reaction, burning, redness and sometimes injury upon their direct application and massaging onto the skin, the carrier oils are not only safe when it comes to the application but also are used to make the essential oils ready for topical application.

What is the use of a Carrier oil?

As the name suggests, the carrier oils are added to the essential oils and other oils/ extracts that are to be applied on to the skin. They dilute them and make them safe for topical application. The term carrier oil is given to these oils keeping in mind the purpose they are being used for, that is, carrying the essential oils from their storage to be used in the topical application. Aloe Vera gel is also used as a carrier for the essential oils.

The body oils, natural lotions, bath oils, creams, lip balms and related moisturizing skin care products including unscented body lotion are also manufactured using the carrier oils or the vegetable oils.

Difference between Essential Oil and Carrier Oil

The essential oils are the product of steam distillation of the root, bark, leaves, flowers. They can also be obtained from any aromatic part of the therapeutic plant which can be evaporated and is characterized by their specific aroma. Over time, the essential oils are known to lose their therapeutic potential and oxidize, however, there is no sign of getting putrid or become rancid of essential oils.

On the other hand, the carrier oil is obtained by the pressing of the fatty parts of the therapeutic plant, nuts, kernel, and seeds. The carrier oils are neither known evaporating nor are they seen imparting the characteristic aroma as strongly and effectively as done by the former, the essential oils. It has been in the knowledge that carrier oils tend to go putrid and rancid with the passage of time.

Carrier oils Degrade, Essential oils Do not.

Choice of a Carrier oil

The carrier oils vary greatly in their properties and therapeutic potential. Thus, the choice of a carrier oil, like an essential oil, for an essential oil depends upon the type of therapeutic treatment or the result required.

The path from an essential oil, to an essential oil and carrier oil or vegetable oil blend to a moisturizing cream or lotion complex, depends upon the choice of carrier oil for the specific therapeutic properties, aroma, color and shelf life of the finished product.

Seems complex? It isn't. Let's break it.

$$\text{Essential oil} \rightarrow \text{essential oil} + \text{carrier oil} \rightarrow \text{Moisturizing cream or lotion}$$

The above equation / process depends upon the choice of carrier oil for

i.   the specific therapeutic properties,

ii.   aroma,

iii.   color

iv.   and shelf life of the finished product.

It was that simple.

Choice of Carrier Oils based on Processing Method

The choice of the type of carrier oil though depends upon the type of therapeutic benefit required. However, the choice of carrier oil based on their processing method should be done very carefully, and preference must be given to the <u>heat-less treatment method</u>.

In this respect, cold pressed, and cold expeller pressed carrier oils should have been utilized and given preference. This ensures that the fatty parts of plants upon pressing have experienced the minimum amount heat possible to convert them into carrier oils. This is done to ensure the quality, nutrient content, and integrity of the vegetable oils.

Other Names of Carrier Oils and the Reason Behind those Names

The term 'Carrier Oil' is confined specifically for the aromatherapy which means that within the practice of aromatherapy, the oils used are named carrier oils. Thus, indicating they have other names outside the boundaries and practice of aromatherapy. The carrier oils, in the field of natural skin care, are named as vegetable oils, base oils and fixed oils with a preference on vegetable oils.

This must be kept in mind that there are base oils or fixed oils that are not vegetable oils, for example, the Emu oil obtained from the emu bird and the fish oil obtained from marine fish do not come under the vegetable oil domain and are not used in aromatherapy. Only those oils that are sourced as a vegetable in nature and are used for aromatherapy are vegetable oils; they are carrier oils in the aromatherapy practice.

List of Carrier oils used in the Aromatherapy

Down below, is the list of carrier oils that are being used in the practice of Aromatherapy in the alphabetical order.

i. Almond Oil
ii. Apricot Kernel Oil
iii. Avocado Oil
iv. Borage Seed Oil
v. Camellia Seed Oil or Tea Oil
vi. Coconut Oil (fractionated)
vii. Coconut Oil (virgin)
viii. Cranberry Seed Oil
ix. Evening Primrose Oil
x. Grapeseed Oil
xi. Hazelnut Oil

xii.   Hemp Seed Oil

xiii. JojobaOil

xiv.   Kukui Nut Oil

xv.   Macadamia Nut Oil

xvi.   Meadowfoam Oil

xvii. Olive Oil

xviii. Peanut Oil

xix.   Pecan Oil

xx.   Pomegranate Seed Oil

xxi.   Rose Hip Oil

xxii. Seabuckthorn Berry Oil

xxiii. Sesame Oil

xxiv. Sunflower Oil

xxv.   Watermelon Seed Oil

We are in search for more if this isn't it. Moreover, how to use them? Stay tuned!

Vegetable Butters as Carrier Oils

Quick check! Are you familiar with Shea Butter and Cocoa Butter?

The vegetable butter though does not come under the category of carrier oils. But their beneficial properties especially those of the Shea Butter and the Cocoa Butter are there to make them lipids. Thus, making them equally useful and beneficial to be used in the practice of Aromatherapy.

Vegetable butter is exactly like the vegetable oils except for their physical appearance at room temperature. The vegetable butter is solid rather than liquid as the vegetable oils at room temperature. The processing of butter is carried out by various methods. One should prefer the cold pressed vegetable butter as a purchasing choice.

Infused Oils or Macerated Oils

Do you know? The infused oil is an advanced form of a carrier oil.

It is a carrier oil infused with herbs. The number of added herbs can vary. The infused oils are also known as macerated oils. The infused oils upon use provide dual benefit,

    i.   the benefit of a carrier oil and

    ii.   the added benefit and therapeutic properties of the infused herbs

The dual properties of a carrier oil and herbs are because the herbs are infused into a carrier oil.

Why Infused Herbs?

This is done in the case of plants having a less aromatic composition that cannot be extracted as an essential oil. The plant is unable to yield an essential oil or related products. However, its therapeutic potential is something for which an added step can be taken. Infusing such herbs into carrier oils not only provide added benefits but make the plant eligible for use in the practice of aromatherapy.

Properties of Infused Oils

The infused oils may have an oily feeling at the touch. This depends on the type of carrier oil used in the manufacturing of infused oils. The infused oils are less concentrated in the sense of aromatic composition, aroma, and strength as compared to the essential oils. Moreover, like carrier oils, with vegetable oil properties and fatty acids, infused oils are also potent to rancidity and can become rancid with the passage of time. Infused are commonly made by using and infusing the herb "Calendula" in the carrier oils.

It is taking energy, Hold on! We are about to get over it. It's a short, good read, please.

The other aromatic ingredients are the other plant products that do not come under aromatherapy oils. They are not used in the holistic aromatherapy, except for Resins. However, they have important therapeutic, health and other uses; which is why their knowledge and identification are extremely important to avoid wrong purchase or end up becoming a fool of marketing. They are

Hydrosols or Floral Water
Resins
Fragrance Oil
Floral Essences

These four will be briefly discussed for better understanding.

Hydrosols or Floral Water

Hydrosols, the remains of steam distillation or hydro distillation that are composed of aromatic waters present in the plants. They are sometimes called as distilled waters, hydrolates, and floral waters as well. The example includes the lavender.

Definition

In the words of the author of book Hydrosols: The Next Aromatherapy, Suzanne Catty, "Hydrosols are the condensate water co-produced during the steam- or hydro-distillation of plant material for aromatherapeutic purposes." (Catty, 2001)

There are expert distillers of hydrosols including the author of the book Harvest to Hydrosol, Ann Harman, who are involved in distilling the plants specifically to produce hydrosols. The resultant hydrosols are extremely beneficial and superior when it comes to their therapeutic benefits and specific aroma.

Production of Hydrosols

Many hydrosols are produced by the distillation used to produce essential oils. In the distillation process. The use of plant matter is responsible for imparting the hydrosols with the specific properties of therapeutic benefits and the water-soluble aromatic compounds. To obtain essential oils, the process of distillation is performed. They are then diluted prior application onto the skin. However, the hydrosols being much gentle in nature than the essential oils need no dilution to be applied on the skin.

Uses of Hydrosols

Hydrosols are generally used in the manufacturing of lotions, fragrances, facial toners, creams and other related skin care products in place of water. They are also added to some water baths while they can be applied directly on the body as a body spray or body cologne.

Also, they can be used to add a beautiful fragrance in a romantic or some special dinner or occasion by simply adding them in finger bowls. One must be aware of the blended essential oils being named as floral waters before purchasing. This requires some research and a little effort to obtain the pure hydrosols.

The **examples** of plants available in the market as hydrosols are Roman Chamomiles, Lavender, Rose, and Neroli.

Resins

Remember the trees we used to tease? Those Gummy trees?

Resins are produced by some trees or types of plants. When a plant that is capable of producing resins gets injured, a thick, semi-solid, sticky substance is produced. Famous **examples** of resins include Myrrh, Frankincense, and Benzoin.

Commercial Collection of Resins

For their commercial collection, the tree or plant is subjected to multiple cuts and injuries to obtain the resins in bulk by encouraging resin production. Natural resins are known to provide numerous therapeutic benefits.

Resins Used Fit and Unfit for Aromatherapy

In the practice of aromatherapy, only the liquid resins extracted by alcohol or solvent extractions are utilized. Because most of the resins produced are thick and sticky and unfit for aromatherapy like Benzoin.

The other two frankincense resins and myrrh are collected in the form of solid chunks. They are then powdered to be used for loose incense, as the powders are incorporated in related incense for obtaining medicinal benefits. This is because the frankincense tears, the small solid chunks of frankincense resins and solid myrrh are not fit for use in the holistic aromatherapy because of their physical condition, that is their resinous form.

How to make Unfit, Fit?

The frankincense and myrrh resins are incorporated in holistic aromatherapy by obtaining their essential oils. After steam distillation of collected myrrh resin and frankincense resin respectively. They are also used in-room fragrance, spiritual therapy, and perfume application.

Fragrance Oil

Short Reminder: We covered them slightly earlier as well. Remember?

It is just a recall to the previously covered topic.

Fragrance oils, potpourri oils or perfume oils are very different from the essential oils. Essential oils are composed of the distilled essence of the plant, the fragrance oils are either the fragrances produced artificially using artificial substances or the product of carrier oil dilution. The fragrance oils cannot reach the aromatic quality and the therapeutic benefits being offered by the essential oils.

However, they are often mistaken as the essential oils because of their packaging and falsified or misleading labeling. Moreover, incomplete labeling also results in the assumption of fragrance oils as the essential oils. Examples are:

    a. Sandalwood Fragrance Oil
    b. Neroli Fragrance Oil

Do not get trapped! Fragrance oils are nowhere near Essential oils.

Floral Essences

What comes to your mind with the word Floral Essence? Essence of Flowers.

Yes, it is.

Production of Floral Essence

Floral Essence is produced by a tedious process. It starts with the addition of flower petals in the spring water. The water containing petal is then basked in the sun to let the flower petals release their essence into the spring water. It can be boiled depending upon the type of effect required. The mixture is then diluted further with the addition of more spring water. Lastly, brandy (alcohol) is added to preserve the floral essence obtained.

Properties of Floral Essence

It is the water used in the homeopathic treatment and not used in typical aromatherapy (though a diluted version is sometimes used). However, it has amazing spiritual properties, like, aiding in combatting the fear of supernatural, eradication of jealousy and selfishness. It adds a positive effect on hopeless, discouraged, impatient, sinful and traumatized people.

Floral Essence has the property of Healing Spiritual Diseases.

Keeping in Mind

- There are Aromatherapy oils and other aromatic ingredients used in or associated to Aromatherapy.
- The Aromatherapy oils include the primary products used in aromatherapy like essential oils, absolutes, CO_2 extracts, carrier oils and infused oils.
- Absolutes are the aromatic plant extracts, obtained by chemical solvent extraction and are more concentrated than essential oils.
- CO_2 extracts are the aromatic plant extracts, obtained by liquefied CO_2 extraction and are better than essential oils.
- Carrier oils are the plant extracts obtained from the fatty portion of the plant and are added to essential oils for use in aromatherapy.
- Infused oils are the carrier oils infused with beneficial herbs and are a recent addition to aromatherapy.
- The other aromatic ingredients are non-oil products that are not used in holistic aromatherapy (except for resins). They have numerous therapeutic and other benefits.
- Hydrosols are the distillation by-product of essential oil production and are used in making lotion and toners. They are used as carriers.
- Resins are the sticky, thick, semi-solid plant products that are used in different aromatherapy practices after passing through various procedures.
- Fragrance oils are the synthetic products and are not used in aromatherapy.

- Floral essence is the plant floral extracts used for healing spiritual complications.

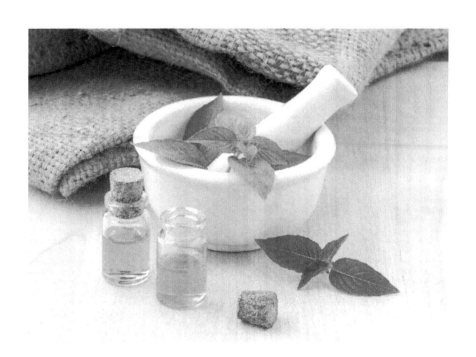

CHAPTER 4

ESSENTIAL OILS USED IN

AROMATHERAPY

AND THEIR IMPORTANCE

Now that you have understood the important concepts and read the information about the Essential oils, Aromatherapy and the oils and ingredients used or linked to Aromatherapy. It is time to know about the essential oils used in aromatherapy at present.

In this chapter, more than 170 essential oils will be discussed briefly. This chapter is what you were waiting for since the start of this book. It is here.

You have reached so far. Good going!

Below is the list of all the essential oil that we will read about in Chapter No. 4 and later in the book as well. These are all the essential oils available at present.

Full A–Z List of Essential Oils

1. Allspice
2. Ambrette Seed
3. Amyris
4. Angelica Root
5. Anise
6. Anise, Star
7. Atlas Cedarwood
8. Balsam, Peru
9. Basil
10. Basil, Holy
11. Bay
12. Bay Laurel
13. Beeswax
14. Benzoin
15. Bergamot
16. Bergamot Mint
17. Black Pepper
18. Blood Orange
19. Blue Cypress
20. Blue Tansy
21. Bois de Rose
22. Boronia
23. Bursera Graveolens
24. Cade
25. Cajeput
26. Camphor, White
27. Cananga
28. Caraway Seed
29. Cardamom
30. Carrot Seed
31. Cassia
32. Catnip/Catmint
33. Cedarwood, Atlas
34. Cedarwood, Virginian
35. Chamomile, German
36. Chamomile, Roman
37. Chocolate Peppermint
38. Cilantro
39. Cinnamon
40. Cistus
41. Citronella
42. Clary Sage
43. Clove Bud
44. Coffee
45. Common Sage
46. Copaiba Balsam
47. Coriander
48. Cornmint
49. Cumin
50. Cypress
51. Cypress, Blue
52. Davana
53. Dill
54. Dalmatian Sage
55. Elemi
56. Eucalyptus Globulus
57. Eucalyptus, Lemon
58. Eucalyptus Radiata
59. Fennel
60. Fir Needle
61. Fragonia
62. Frankincense

63.	Galbanum	99.	Marjoram
64.	Geranium	100.	May Chang
65.	Geranium, Rose	101.	Melissa
66.	German Chamomile	102.	Mullein
67.	Ginger	103.	Myrrh
68.	Grapefruit	104.	Myrrh, Sweet
69.	Gurjum Balsam	105.	Myrtle
70.	Helichrysum	106.	Myrtle, Lemon
71.	Hemlock	107.	Neroli
72.	Ho Leaf	108.	Niaouli
73.	Ho Wood	109.	Nutmeg
74.	Holy Basil	110.	Oakmoss
75.	Hops	111.	Olibanum
76.	Hyssop	112.	Opoponax
77.	Immortelle	113.	Orange, Bitter
78.	Jasmine	114.	Orange, Blood
79.	Juniper Berry	115.	Orange, Sweet
80.	Kanuka	116.	Oregano
81.	Kunzea	117.	Palmarosa
82.	Labdanum	118.	Palo Santo
83.	Laurel Leaf	119.	Parsley
84.	Lavandin	120.	Patchouli
85.	Lavandula abrialis	121.	Pepper, Black
86.	Lavender	122.	Pepper, Pink
87.	Lavender, Spike	123.	Peppermint
88.	Lemon	124.	Peppermint, Chocolate
89.	Lemon Balm		
90.	Lemon Eucalyptus	125.	Peru Balsam
91.	Lemongrass	126.	Petitgrain
92.	Lemon Myrtle	127.	Pimento Berry/Leaf
93.	Lemon Tea Tree		
94.	Lime	128.	Pine, Pinyon
95.	Linden Blossom	129.	Pine, Scotch
96.	Mandarin	130.	Pink Pepper
97.	Mandravasarotra	131.	Ravensara
98.	Manuka	132.	Ravintsara

133. Rock Rose
134. Roman Chamomile
135. Rose
136. Rosemary
137. Rosewood
138. Sage, Clary
139. Sage, Common
140. Sage, Dalmatian
141. Sage, Spanish
142. Sandalwood
143. Saro
144. Scotch Pine
145. Spearmint
146. Spike Lavender
147. Spikenard
148. Spruce
149. Spruce, Hemlock
150. Star Anise
151. Sweet Myrrh
152. Sweet Orange
153. Tagetes
154. Tangerine
155. Tansy, Blue
156. Tea Tree, Common
157. Tea Tree, Lemon
158. Tea Tree, New Zealand
159. Thyme
160. Tobacco
161. Tuberose
162. Tulsi
163. Vanilla
164. Vetiver
165. Violet Leaf
166. Virginian Cedarwood
167. White Camphor
168. Wintergreen
169. Yarrow
170. Ylang Ylang
171. Yuzu

We will discuss the most important 91 among them.

91 A-Z Descriptions
of the Most Important Essential Oils

A few of the prominent properties and health benefits of these Essential Oils are mentioned under each Essential Oil's description. Some provide a wide range of benefits while some are used for specific health conditions. Read them out and diversify your knowledge.

Let's get started!

A

1. Allspice Essential Oil

Allspice Essential Oil is a good analgesic, anesthetic, antioxidant, relaxant, stimulant, antiseptic tonic. It is used to relieve pain and induce numbness. Allspice is used to add color to the skin. It is also used to relax both mind and body.

2. Ambrette Seed Essential Oil

Ambrette seed essential oil is an unmistakable aromatic oil with a beautiful Aroma. Ambrette seed oil contains a lot of palmitic acid and is popular for treating anxiety, fatigue, stress, cramp, headaches, indigestion and more. Also, interestingly, it is often considered a powerful aphrodisiac due to its intoxicating scent and calming properties hence making it a great choice for aromatherapy and relaxing bath.

3. Amyris Essential Oil

Amyris Essential Oil, also known as Indies Sandalwood or the West Indian Rosewood. This essential oil originates from the West Indies, specifically in Haiti. Due to its soft aroma and long-lasting fragrance, it is often used as a "Fixating agent" in perfumes to increase the fragrance's life. Health benefits include a relaxant, skin cleanser & toner along with anti-depressant.

4. Angelica Root Essential Oil

It is a diuretic, stimulant, hepatic, anti-spasmodic, digestive stomachic, expectorant, and tonic. Angelica Root Essential Oil is used to increase urine, relaxes spasms. It is good for liver, stomach and improves digestion. It relieves the body from gases, obstructed menstruation and removes toxins. It cures nervous disorders, purifies the blood, reduces fever, promotes perspiration and expels catarrh and phlegm. Angelica Essential Oil is also used in toning the body.

5. Anise Essential Oil

Anise Essential Oil is anti-epileptic, antiseptic, antirheumatic, anti-hysteric, decongestant, insecticide. This essential oil is used to treat epilepsy, spasms, rheumatism, hysteria, arthritis. It provides protection from septic attack, insects like worms and lice. It relieves the body from congestion and aids in breathing. It acts as a sedative and induces sleep. Releasing gases, improving digestion and removing toxins are some other benefits practitioners acquire from Anise essential oil.

6. Atlas Cedarwood Essential Oil

Cedarwood essential oil is extracted from the leftover steam-distilled wood chips and sawdust used for construction and furniture making. The Atlas Cedarwood has a slightly sharper aroma as compared to Virginian cedarwood. It is also considered much safer to use. It has remarkable antiseptic and antipruritic properties for eczema, skin and scalp problems.

Due to its astringent properties, it is also suggested to be used as a remedy for acne, dandruff, and oily skin. It has a calming effect which helps in overcoming nervous tension, stress, and anxiety. This essential oil is extremely beneficial for respiratory problems. They include chronic coughs and bronchitis. Cedarwood Essential Oil help loosen and clear the accumulated mucus. The antiseptic properties of this essential oil aid in treating urinary tract infections. Though, the changes are mild, yet, effective in the case of circulatory and lymphatic stimulation. It helps in combating the fluid retention and cellulite removal.

B

7. Balsam Essential Oil or Peru Essential Oil

Balsam Essential Oil is being used for topical wound treatment and infections in certain parts of the world for ages. In India, it is also used to stop excessive bleeding as it promotes wound healing. Along with being used in Food industry as an additive, it also plays a useful part in pharmaceutical preparations and perfumery. Balsam oils are mildly antiseptic and can be used as disinfectants.

8. Basil Essential Oil

The Basil Essential oil acts as an analgesic, anti-spasmodic. It has carminative, ophthalmic and antibacterial properties as well. The Basil Essential oil helps in resolving digestion, blood circulation, and respiratory issues. It eases the pain, omits vomiting and releases stress. It also helps in combating infections.

9. Holy Basil Essential Oil

Holy basil (Ocimum tenuiflorum) is different from the casual basil used in marinara sauce or Thai herbs. Commonly known as Tulsi, it has a history of treatment for eye diseases and ringworms. Holy Basil's fresh flower oil is good for bronchitis, leaves and seed oil for malaria, whole plant for the treatment of Gut discomfort like diarrhea, nausea, vomiting, etc. Eczema ointments are also prepared form basil extracts.

10. Bay Essential Oil

Bay Essential Oil is used commonly as an antibiotic, antiseptic, anti-neuralgic, analgesic, anti-spasmodic properties. It also possesses insecticidal, sedative and tonic properties. Bay Essential Oil inhibits microbial growth, relieves pain, relaxes spasms. It is used by some practitioners to cure neuralgia pain. Bay Essential Oil increases appetite, prevents hair loss, tightens muscles and gums. It provides protection against septic attacks

Bay Essential Oil treats hemorrhage, relieves obstructed menstruation, reduces fever and promotes bile secretion. Along with sedating nerve afflictions and inflammations, it acts as an insect killer and repellant. It increases perspiration, enhances the stomach activity and improves health by eliminating toxins from the body.

11. Beeswax

Besides its tremendous uses in everyday life, Beeswax is an excellent addition to cosmetic products, for many notable reasons. It creates a barrier to help seal the moisture into the skin. This is especially beneficial in lip chap during the dry winter months. This barrier also helps to protect the skin from environmental toxins and irritants.

Unlike petroleum jelly, which is used in a large variety of beauty products, beeswax will not "suffocate" the skin, but rather, allow it to breathe while still providing a protective barrier.

Beeswax helps to thicken homemade cosmetics and lotions because it is solid at room temperature and has a relatively high melting point of 147 degrees Fahrenheit. This is especially helpful in recipes that include high amounts of coconut oil, which has a low melting point, or other oils that are liquid at room temperature.

Beeswax also has Vitamin A, which improves hydration to the skin and promotes cell regeneration.

12. Benzoin Essential Oil

Benzoin Essential Oil provides amazing health benefits as it acts as an antidepressant, antidiuretic, and disinfectant. It is anti-inflammatory, antiseptic, anti-rheumatic and relaxant sedative. Benzoin Essential Oil also provides deodorant, cordial and carminative properties.

Benzoin Essential Oil uplifts moods, fights depression, and hopelessness. It is used to get rid of the body's building gases that cause severe discomfort. It reduces body order, promotes relaxation, cures infections and removes body toxins by promoting their removal via urination.

Strengthening of gums, reduction in hemorrhaging while improved circulation and curing inflammation are added benefits. A bonus is Benzoin Essential Oil's property to aid in curing arthritis and calming anxiety while relieving tension.

13. Bergamot Essential Oil

The properties of Bergamot Essential Oil include antibiotic, sedative, antiseptic, analgesic, and anti-spasmodic. It acts as an antidepressant, deodorant, digestive and disinfectant in nature. The Bergamot Essential Oil relieves spasms, removes body odor, suppresses pain, fights depression and improves mood. It aids in healing cuts and scars. It also promotes efficient digestive mechanism in the body.

14. Bergamot Mint

Bergamot Mint, along with being a magical relaxant, it works great as an inhaler along with rosewood oil. It can also be used effectively as an anti-inflammatory as a remedy for insect bites or bee stings. It helps reduce the pain and itching.

15. Birch Essential Oil

Birch Essential Oil is an antidepressant, disinfectant, stimulant, tonic & analgesic. It has the properties of an anti-rheumatic and anti-arthritic agent. Moreover, Birch Essential Oil is a detoxifier, a diuretic, an antiseptic, a germicide, an insecticide, and an astringent.

Birch Essential Oil provides the health benefits of fighting with depression. It protects the wounds from sepsis and reduces pain. Birch Essential Oil promotes urination, kills insects and germs, reduces fever, and helps in purifying the blood.

16. Bitter Almond Essential Oil

The traditional properties of Birch Almond Essential Oil bactericide, fungicide, germicide, and vermifuge. It acts as an anesthetic, sedative, diuretic, antispasmodic and an anti-toxin. The Bitter Almond Essential Oil is used to cure hydrophobia as well.

It is used to kill worms, germs including bacteria and fungi. Bitter Almond Essential Oil aids in reducing fever and inflammation. It promotes sedation, causes numbness and acts as a desensitizing agent. It increases urination to help remove excess toxins from the body. Bitter Almond Essential Oil has intoxicating effects. It aids in curing spasms and hydrophobia.

17. Black Pepper Essential Oil

Black Pepper Essential Oil is an anti-spasmodic, anti-arthritic, anti-rheumatic, anti-bacterial, and an anti-oxidant by nature. It also has digestive, carminative, diaphoretic properties.

This particular essential oil increases perspiration, removes toxins and gases, acting as a purgative and promotes digestion. It also helps in curing spasms, treating arthritis and rheumatism. For this, toxins including uric acid are removed from the body. It fights premature aging and inhibits bacterial growth. It is also known to neutralize the free radicals present in the body that damage it in countless ways.

18. Blood Orange Essential Oil

The blood orange essential oil, derived by cold compression from its peel, has a fruity, citrus scent which smells great. Therapeutic properties are included but not limited to Anti-inflammation, anti-spasmodic, antiseptic, carminative tendencies. Along with being an effective diuretic, it is also a highly recommended sedative.

19. Blue Tansy Essential Oil

Blue Tansy also known as Moroccan Chamomile oil is one of the rare essential oils. It is extremely hard to get a pure and genuine extract due to its holistic aroma-therapeutic applications. It is royal blue in color and has sweet and slightly floral aroma with a hint of camphor. It is a doctors' most frequently recommended anti-inflammatory, anti-histamine, and anti-allergen. It works miraculously well for fungal infections.

20. Bois de Rose

Bois de Rose has miraculous abilities for skin treatments and marks. It has remarkable action on skin and removes wrinkles tightening skin and removes stretch marks and acne marks. It is also used as a toner for lightening skin tone and vanish signs of aging specifically caused by the flabby/loose skin after severe illness or weight loss.

21. Boldo Essential Oil

Boldo Essential Oil has the properties of anti-rheumatic, anti-inflammatory and an antiseptic agent. It is diuretic, digestive and hepatic in nature. Boldo Essential Oil is a narcotic, an insecticide, a stimulant and a vermifuge in additional properties.

Boldo Essential Oil is known to treat rheumatism, reduce inflammation and provide protection against septic attack. It can treat arthritis, promote bile secretion, increase urination and facilitate the process of digestion. Boldo Essential Oil promotes the removal of toxins. It keeps the liver healthy. Boldo Essential Oil is responsible for repelling and killing insects.

22. Boronia Essential Oil

Boronia oil is being used as an uplifting, refreshing and energizing agent for many years in different parts of the world. It is famous for its rich intense and long-lasting aroma hence being the perfect choice for quality perfumes. Additionally, it is also used as an excellent flavor enhancer for berry and citrus formulations. Medicinally famous for antidepressants, stress relief, and aphrodisiacs.

23. Buchu Essential Oil

Buchu Essential Oil is anti-rheumatic, anti-septic and anti-arthritic in nature. It is a carminative, a diuretic, a digestive, a tonic and an insecticide in its properties.

It treats rheumatism, removes gases, aids in arthritis treatment and provides protection against septic attack. Buchu Essential Oil facilitates digestion, removes toxins and increases urination. It is known for killing insects and repelling them. It also tones up the body.

24. Bursera Graveolens Essential Oil

Palo Santo Oil or "Holy Wood" is known to purify and cleanse the aura from evil spirits and negative energies. It is regarded as a spiritual oil and has very revitalizing benefits. It is known for immune system stimulation and inflammation remedies. Bursera Graveolens boost immunity which strengthens body's defense against inflammations and antigens.

C

25. Cade Essential Oil

Cade oil has antimicrobial, antiseptic and fungicidal applications and has been used for many years in the history traced back to as early as the nineteenth century for soothing skin and scalp irritations such as eczema, dandruff, and psoriasis. Cade oil has pleasant feel due to its strong woody and smoky aroma.

26. Cajuput Essential Oil

Cajuput Essential Oil has antiseptic properties, and it is used as a cosmetic. Other properties include that of an insecticide, a bactericide, and a vermifuge. It acts as a decongestant, anti-neuralgic, analgesic and an anti-spasmodic.

Cajuput Essential Oil is known to provide protection against wounds to prevent them from becoming a septic. This oil kills insects, bacteria and worms, it is involved in skin care, and cures congestion by easing breathing. The Cajuput Essential Oil is known to reduce pain and fever, cure spasm and cough. It can relieve neuralgic pain, remove gases and stimulate secretions to induce nerve response. It increases perspiration, tones the body, relieves obstructed blood by regulating menstruation.

27. Calamus Essential Oil

Calamus Essential Oil is a circulatory stimulant, cephalic and memory boosting properties. This essential oil is anti-spasmodic, anti-rheumatic, stimulant, nervine and a tranquilizer in nature.

It can treat arthritis and rheumatism. Calamus Essential Oil inhibits microbial growth, relaxes spasm and is involved in boosting memory and brain activity. Moreover, it brings good to blood and lymph circulation, it induces sleep and can cure nervous disorders.

28. Camomile Essential Oil

Camomile is an essential oil which has amazing anti-allergenic abilities. It helps cure acne by removing toxins and cleaning skin and sebaceous glands by induced sweating. It also works as a diuretic and cleans up the urinary system, increasing kidney function which results in excessive urination. Camomile is also known to cure viral infections like measles, mumps, etc. German Camomile is believed to help prevent atherosclerosis by working as a vasoconstrictor and reducing blood pressure.

29. Camphor, White Essential Oil

Camphor essential oil or Cinnamomum camphora is a powerful oil with a wide range of excellent health benefits. While the essential oil is usually referred to as camphor oil, it is actually only white camphor oil that can be used medicinally.

It possesses various health benefits and properties including decongestant, antispasmodic, anesthetic, sedative and anti-inflammatory properties. Camphor oil is used as an ingredient in many decongestant balms and soothing cold rubs like tiger balm and Vicks vaporub.

Benefits include muscle pain and spasm relaxant, and effective against rheumatism and arthritis.

30. Carrot Seed Essential Oil

The carrot seed essential oil has a woody aroma and is golden-yellow in color. The health benefits of this oil are many: Its anticarcinogenic properties help in curing cancers of the stomach, mouth, prostate, etc. Carrot seed oil helps flush out toxic substances like bile and uric acid from the body by increasing urination, as it is a natural diuretic.

31. Clary Sage Essential Oil

The essential oil is a leaf and bud oil. It has a clean, refreshing scent that you can use as a skin balm or gently inhale as part of an aromatherapy treatment.

Aromatherapy uses the power of scent to calm the mind and reduce feelings of anxiety. Your olfactory system directly affects the part of your brain that regulates emotion. That's why what you smell can trigger memories and elicit feelings, both negative and positive.

One component of clary sage oil is sclareol, which mimics the effects of estrogen in the body. For this reason, clary sage may be effective at reducing some of the symptoms of menopause. Some research suggests that diluted clary sage oil applied to the bottoms of the feet can reduce hot flashes. It is also known to reduce menstrual cramps when added to the cream.

32. Coffee Essential Oil

Coffee essential oil has antioxidant properties and can help enhance liver function and lower the risk of liver cirrhosis. It can also be used in case of a blocked nose. It can help clear blocked nasal passages. Nausea can also be treated by using coffee oil instead of OTC medication. One of its many uses is it keep insects at bay hence, can be used as mosquito repellent.

33. Cypress Essential Oil

Cypress oil works as Antiseptic in fast healing of wounds, itching, eczema, and psoriasis. It has effective Antispasmodic properties and effects by relaxing muscles and nerves will give you quick relief of cramps and muscle spasms. Due to its pleasant fragrance, it is used in Deodorants and is great for eliminating body odor. For aiding kidney functions, it works as a Diuretic by increasing urination which will help you lose weight and remove unneeded toxins in your body.

It is a strong sedative and also helps reduce Anxiety when inhaled as aromatherapy and an Antidepressant, i.e., it has a positive impact on the psychology of a person.

D

34. Davana Essential Oil

This oil is used as an antiseptic, antidepressant and disinfectant. It also acts as a relaxant, and it is antiviral. It uplifts the mood and fights against depression. So, it relaxes mind and body and also protects wounds from becoming septic. It provides relief from unregulated menstrual cycle by regulating them.

35. Dill Essential Oil

It is used as a digestive, antispasmodic and stomachic. It gives healthy digestion and eliminates the excess gases from the body. It increases perspiration and the secretion of milk.

E

36. Elemi Essential Oil

It is mostly used as a tonic and as an analgesic. It is very helpful in relieving pain and protects against septic. It increases the health of the body and muscle tone.

37. Eucalyptus Essential Oil

It can be used as a deodorant, anti-inflammatory, anti-bacterial and antispasmodic. it is also used for the treatment

of muscle pain, respiratory problem, diabetes, wounds, and
fever.

F

38. Fennel Essential Oil

This oil is used as an aperitif, stimulant, vermifuge, and
expectorant. It increases appetite and urination. It also
purifies the blood and regulates the menstruation cycle.
This oil is good for the stomach as it defends from
constipation. And it also defends the body from cough and
cold.

39. Frankincense Essential Oil

It is used as an astringent, cicatrizant, uterine and sedative.
It heals scars and keeps the cells healthy. This oil also fights
with infections and provide good health to the uterus. It
increases urination and promotes digestion.

G

40. Galbanum Essential Oil

It is traditionally used as a detoxifier, vulnerary, and a
circulatory stimulant. It improves skin health and increases
blood circulation. This oil also eases breathing and kills
insects. It speedily heals wounds and removes toxins from
the body.

41. Geranium Essential Oil

It is used as a hemostatic, styptic and hemostatic. Its qualities include it is used to heal scars and stop the body odor. It kills intestinal worms and tones up the body. It induces tightening in the gums of muscles and skin.

42. Ginger Essential Oil

Ginger essential oil is used as bactericidal, stimulant and febrifuge. This oil is known to stop vomiting and promote sweating. It also improves brain quality and function of the memory. It helps to remove body toxins and is known to break body fever. It also cures pain and protects wounds from becoming septic.

43. Grapefruit Essential Oil

This oil acts as an antidepressant, tonic and lymphatic. It is used to fight infections. It reduces depression and uplifts moods and spirits.

H

44. Helichrysum Essential Oil

This oil is an anticoagulant, antimicrobial, antiseptic and fungicidal. This essential oil is used to fight against allergies. It is good for the health of the nervous system and maintains the fluidity of blood. It reduces healed scars and various types of inflammation. It stimulates urination and regeneration of new cells.

45. Hyssop Essential Oil

This essential oil is an antirheumatic, carminative and cicatrizant. It is hypertensive and an expectorant. Its health benefits are decreasing phlegm and coughs. It is good for reducing fever and stress. It also increases the blood pressure and increase urination.

J

46. Jasmine Essential Oil

Jasmine essential oil is an aphrodisiac, expectorant, and galactagogue. Its properties are sedative and cicatrizant. Jasmine essential oil health benefits include it cures sexual dysfunctions and increase breast milk. This oil relieves labor pain and eases in the delivery of babies.

47. Juniper Essential Oil

This oil is known to be an antispasmodic, sudorific and depurative. Juniper essential oil cures arthritis and rheumatism. It also purifies the blood and stimulates body functions. This oil makes the gums stronger, and it also stops hemorrhaging. It brings color to the skin and quickly heals wounds.

L

48. Lavandin Essential Oil

It is mainly used as an analgesic, nervine and expectorant. It commonly fights against depression. It reduces pain and strengthens the nervous system. It clears phlegm and heals the after marks scars.

49. Lavender Essential Oil

The properties of lavender essential oil are that it induces sleep and makes a person calm. It is anti-inflammatory and antifungal. This oil is also beneficial for the treatment of nervous system issues, insomnia, and respiratory system disorder. It is also used for the care of hair and skin. It also treats the health of the immune system and indigestion.

50. Lemmon Essential Oil

The properties of this oil are that it is restorative and hemostatic. Lemmon essential oil is febrifuge and antiviral. This oil protects the body from bacterial and inhibiting viral growth. It also stops hair loss and uplifts the skin. This oil cures fever and fights with infections.

51. Lemongrass Essential Oil

Lemongrass essential oil is an antipyretic, antimicrobial and analgesic. It also acts as a deodorant and is insecticidal and tonic. Lemongrass inhibits microbial growth. This oil kills bacteria and reduces body odor. It stops fungal infections and soothes inflammation and also strengthens the nerves.

52. Lime Essential Oil

This oil is hemostatic and tonic. It protects from viral infection and wounds from becoming septic. Lime essential oil stops hemorrhaging and boosts both health and appetite.

M

53. Mandarin Essential Oil

It is used as a depurative, nervous relaxant and hepatic. Mandarin essential oil increase blood and lymph circulation. This oil is good for the liver and promotes the growth and regeneration of the cells. This essential oil is good for toning up the body. This oil purifies the blood and soothes nervous afflictions.

54. Manuka Essential Oil

This essential oil acts as an anti-dandruff and antidotes for the stings and the bites of insects. This oil is an antihistaminic, cicatrizant and cytophylactic. It is commonly used to counter venomous bites. It sedates inflammation and checks the production of histamine. It also clears spots and scars very quickly. This essential oil reduces allergic symptoms.

55. Marjoram Essential Oil

This essential oil is an anaphrodisiac, cephalic, cordial and diuretic. This oil can act as a laxative, nervine, vasodilator, and emmenagogue. The health benefits of the marjoram essential oil are commonly chosen for the treatment. This oil cures cramp, eliminates spasm, and reduces pain. It opens the obstructed periods, and it also relaxes and widens blood vessels.

56. Melissa Essential Oil

Melissa essential oil is used as an antibacterial, hypotensive and a diaphoretic. This essential oil is commonly used to cure nervous disorder. It inhibits the bacteria while removing gas and toxins from the body and increase perspiration. It boosts up the health of the immune system and lowers blood pressure.

57. Mugwort Essential Oil

Mugwort essential oil is used as a stimulant, cordial and emmenagogue. This essential oil helps in digestion and stimulates systematic functions. It also kills the intestinal worms and maintains the uterine health.

58. Mullein Essential Oil

This essential oil is used as a tranquilizer, relaxant, and disinfectant. This essential oil is used to protect from wounds and relieve pain. It also expels both catarrh and phlegm from the body. Furthermore, it induces sleep and relaxes the body and mind.

59. Mustard Essential Oil

Mustard essential oil is used as an appetizer, irritant, hair revitalizer, and insect repellant. This essential oil is used to reduce hair fall and boost the hair growth. It is also used to stimulate discharges, increases fungal growth and appetite. It also helps to cure rheumatism and increases perspiration.

60. Myrrh Essential Oil

This essential oil is used as an anti-catarrhal, astringent and expectorant. Myrrh essential oil is used as an immune and circulatory booster. This essential oil is traditionally used for tightening muscles and gums. It is also used to curb microbial growth and stimulates discharges. It is good for the health of stomach, and it also protects from arthritis. This oil improves circulation of blood and protects from diseases.

61. Myrtle Essential Oil

Myrtle essential oil is used as a sedative and an expectorant.

94

It is used to protect from ulcers transforming into serious infections. It reduces the odor of body and stops hemorrhaging.

N

62. Neroli Essential Oil

This essential oil is a cicatrizant, emollient and antispasmodic. It is helpful in fading scars speedily and after marks and promotes the growth of cells. This oil soothes from inflammation and anxiety.

63. Niaouli Essential Oil

This oil is used as a balsamic and decongestant. Niaouli essential oil is used to clear spots and decreases congestion. It eases breathing and inhibits bacterial growth.

64. Nutmeg Essential Oil

This essential oil is considered as anti-parasitic and antiemetic. It is used as a prostaglandin, cardiac and laxative. It helps to protect wounds from developing sepsis. It counters premature aging and stops enlargement of the prostate. This oil is used to enhance libido and improves the health of the heart.

O

65. Oakmoss Essential Oil

Oakmoss essential oil is used as a demulcent. This essential oil helps in restoring health.

66. Orange Essential Oil

This essential oil is a cholagogue and diuretic. It is used to cure sexual dysfunction and enhance libido. It increases urination, discharges, and secretions from glands. It is also used to tone up the general health of the immune system.

67. Oregano Essential Oil

Oregano essential oil is an antiviral, anti-allergic and antibacterial. It is mostly used to inhibit bacterial, peracetic and fungal infections. It heals the damages done by the oxidation.

P

68. Palma Rosa Essential Oil

It is used as a bactericide, cytophylactic, hydration balm and febrifuge. This essential oil protects from sepsis, promotes regeneration of cells, and facilitates digestion.

69. Parsley Essential Oil

Parsley essential oil is an antarthritic, hypotensive and depurative. This oil is essential in reducing blood pressure and clears the bowels. It soothes fever and removes toxins from the body.

69. Patchouli Essential Oil

This essential oil is an antiphlogistic, fungicide and insecticide. It is also known for increasing urination and to stop hemorrhaging.

70. Pennyroyal Essential Oil

This oil is a decongestant, ant hysteric, stomachic and an astringent. This oil is mostly used by physicians. Pennyroyal essential oil is used to clear congestion and also clear the blood. It is also used to make menstruation regular.

71. Peppermint Essential Oil

It is used as an antigalactogogue, cholagogue, hepatic, vasoconstrictor and cephalic. This oil is used to induce numbness. It also reduces the milk flow and induces firmness in the muscles and promote bile discharge. It is also good for memory health and brain. Furthermore, peppermint oil slight contraction of blood vessels.

72. Petitgrain Essential Oil

Petitgrain oil is a sedative and an antiseptic. It is commonly used to relax spasms and reduce nervous afflictions.

73. Pimento Essential Oil

This oil is a rubefacient, anesthetic, and an anti-oxidant. Pimento essential oil traditionally fights with premature aging. It brings coloration to the skin and increases tone.

74. Pine Essential Oil

Pine essential oil is used as a diuretic, energizing and an aromatic substance. Pine oil is commonly used in cosmetics and helps in skin care. It relieves mental fatigue and urinary tract infections.

R

75. Ravensara Essential Oil

It is well-known as an aphrodisiac, analgesic and for tonic compound. Ravensara oil relief from microbial growth. It increases subsequent removal of toxins and catarrh.

76. Rose Essential Oil

Rose essential oil is used for uterine oil substance. Rose oil promotes discharges and secretion. It is good for stomach and cures constipation.

77. Rosemary Essential Oil

Rosemary oil is excellent for stimulating the hair growth. It is carminative and an analgesic substance. It is helpful in terms of mouth, hair and skin care. It relief bronchial asthma, headache, flatulence, and indigestion.

78. Rue Essential Oil

It is utilized as a deterrent for various nervous infection. It also neutralizes the effect of poison and removal of uric acid. Furthermore, it relieves hysteresis and epileptic attacks and keeps the nerves steady.

S

79. Sage Essential Oil

Sage oil is normally considered as an expectorant. It increases the production of bile and boosts the systematic functions.

80. Sandalwood Essential Oil

It is used as a memory booster and hypotensive. It keeps skin smooth and free from infections.

81. Spearmint Essential Oil

It is a stimulating substance, antiseptic and carminative. It heals general tear and wear.

82. Spikenard Essential Oil

Spikenard oil is a uterine substance and an antibacterial. It is traditionally used to sedate inflammation while restoring uterine health.

T

83. Tagetes Essential Oil

It is an antimicrobial and an antibiotic. This oil is used to inhibit microbial and other parasitic growth.

84. Tangerine Essential Oil

Tangerine oil is used as a tonic substance. It is also used to purify the blood, promote the growth of cells and reduce nervous order.

85. Tansy Essential Oil

Tansy oil is an antiviral, vermifuge substance and a hormone stimulant. It is used as the curb to produce histamine.

86. Tarragon Essential Oil

Tarragon oil is a circulatory agent, and it is used to treats rheumatism.

87. Tea Tree Essential Oil

This oil is antibacterial, balsamic, sudorific in nature and promoting absorption of nutrients.

88. Thuja Essential Oil

This essential oil is an insect repellant, rubefacient, and an emmenagogue. It increases urination and expels catarrh and phlegm.

89. Thyme Essential Oil

This oil is an antiseptic, bechic and a vermifuge substance. This essential oil helps to cure chest infections and good for heart health.

90. Tuberose Essential Oil

Tuberose oil is used as a warming substance. This oil is used to enhance libido.

V

91. Vanilla Essential Oil

Vanilla oil is a relaxing substance and tranquilizing. It is also used to neutralize the effects of free radicals.

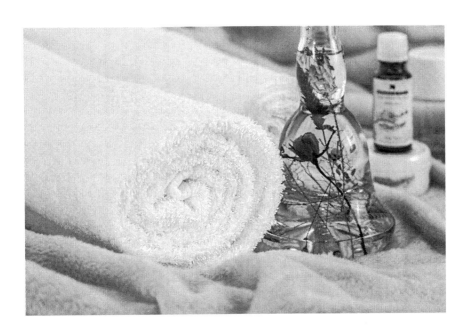

CHAPTER 5

PERFORMING AROMATHERAPY

Now that you have gone through all the initial details, it is time to move on to the most important part. In this Chapter, you will get the answer to your long-asked question.

How to perform an Aromatherapy?

We know, you were longing for it for long. But you know, there is the right time for everything. It is the time!

Aromatherapy can be performed in different ways using different products and carriers. The list below will provide you a brief idea about How to perform an Aromatherapy?

Aromatherapy Massage

    Using Carrier Oils

    Using Toners and Lotions

Aromatherapy Baths

Aromatherapy Spritzer

Steam Inhalation

Inhalation Aromatherapy

    Direct Inhalation

    Direct Palm Inhalation

    Direct Bottle Inhalation

    Cotton Balls

    Smelling Salts

    Inhaler Tubes

Ingestion Aromatherapy

Aromatherapy Massage

The massage and the body oil is basically the combination of one or more than one vegetable including herbal oils with the essential oils. Massages are generally helpful in reducing stress, and it also helps to relieve pain.

Using Carrier Oils

The massage through carrier oil is mostly used in pregnancy and childbirth. The dilution recommended for infants is 5-1% i-e 3-6 drops of the essential oil per ounce of the carrier. So, for the adults, it is 2.5-10% dilution 15-60 drops of the essential oil per ounce of the carrier. The carrier helps to relax and soothes the nervous system. It enhances immunity and relieves migraine. It also treats strains and repetitive movement injuries.

Using Toners and Lotions

The unscented facial creams and body lotions add in essential oils to create a facial oil also using a variety of herbal or vegetable oils. For the sensitive skin of adult's dilution is recommended to be 5-1% i-e 3-6 drops per ounce and for the healthy skin 1-2.5% i-e 6-15 drops per ounce. It helps to support and enhance the immune cells of the skin and enhances wound healing. It encourages hydration of the skin and influences slow aging. This toner also aids the process of detoxification of the skin.

Aromatherapy Baths

This aromatherapy bath helps reduce pain and stiffness mix 2-12 drops which depend upon the essential oil into a teaspoon of a dispersing agent like a natural bath gel. Stir it just before entering the water. It would not disperse into the water and make the bathing tub slippery. It improves the tone and health of the skin. It also alleviates muscular aches, tension, and pain. This therapy enhances lymph circulation and local circulations.

Aromatherapy Spritzer

This therapy is the combination of both essential oils and water. A dispersant like solubol is used to diffuse essential oil in the water. Aromatic spritzer is also used as a room freshener to energize and uplift it. It is also used in esthetic practice for example if it is sprayed on the face cradles it keeps the respiratory passages clear.

Steam Inhalation

Put 3-7 drops of essential oil into boiling water. Some essential oils to be considered are eucalyptus, lemon, and tea tree oil. Cover the head with the towel and take a breath from the nose while the eyes should be closed. It enhances respiratory function and helps in sinus infections.

Aromatherapy can also be done through inhalation. There are different types of inhalation but have almost similar benefits. It purifies and improves the air quality. It also helps in reducing stress and anxiety.

Direct Inhalation

This type of inhalation referred to sniffing an essential oil directly from the bottle. It can also be inhaled through dipping cotton ball and handkerchief into the bottle. The process of direct inhalation is employed for relieving the emotional distress. It is also a very supportive therapy used for the relief of respiratory congestion and provides relief in other respiratory ailments. It is also used for the better effects on the nervous system.

Direct Palm Inhalation

Direct palm inhalation is referred to a technique in which sniffing or inhaling an essential oil or the synergy directly from the palm of your hand. This type of inhalation is mostly utilized to relieve the emotional distress as well as uplift and transforms the one's consciousness. It also relief other respiratory ailments and is used to relax and breath.

Direct Bottle Inhalation

This type of technique is done through creating a synergy which is an undiluted essential oil i-e utilizing almost 3-5 essential oils and placed in a bottle. For deep inhalation, take a client waft bottle under the nose. It can be done up to 3-4 times a day or as needed.

Cotton Balls

Cotton ball inhalation could be done by placing 2-4 drops of essential oil or synergy on a tissue or a cloth. Hold that piece of cloth in your palm and take a deep inhalation up to 2-3 times through the nose. If you are using a cotton ball, then gently waft the cotton ball under the client's nose. This technique is done for 2-3 times a day or as needed.

Smelling Salts

This technique is done by creating a synergy of 20-30 drops by utilizing 3-5 essential oils. Place it in a 1/3 ounce and 10 ml bottle. The remaining part of the bottle is filled with either a fine or a coarse sea salt. Take the client waft bottle under the nose during deep inhalations. Smelling salt can be done 3-4 times a day or as needed.

Inhaler Tubes

The inhaler tube is designed using 100% essential oil or oils which are saturated on a cotton pad. Choose up to 2-3 essential oils whose work is based upon specific purpose. 15-20 drops of essential oil are added depending on the quantity required for each of the essential oil. Place drops of essential oils in a small bowl or a cup then place pad from inhaler into the ball to absorb all the essential oils. Use the tweezers to move pad around a bit and then remove the pad with the tweezers and place in the inhaler tube. Finally, close the inhaler tube, and now it's ready to use. Inhaler tubes are commonly used to relieve stress and nausea. Support healthy breathing and hormonal balance. It also reduces nasal congestion and uplifts the mood.

Ingestion Aromatherapy

Ingestion aromatherapy can be done via oral intake of Essential oils. This particular aromatherapy cannot be performed unless advised by the Aromatherapy Practitioner.

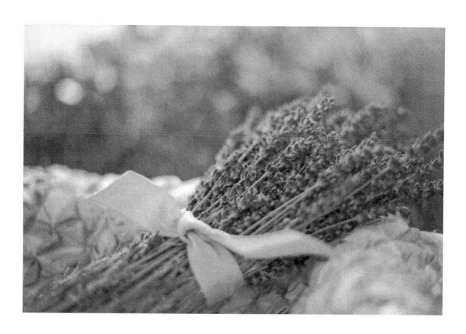

CHAPTER 6

HEALTH COMPLICATIONS AND THEIR

CORRESPONDING ESSENTIAL OILS FOR

AROMATHERAPY

Now that we are done with understanding Essential oils, Aromatherapy oils, and have read almost all in use of Essential oils with the situation they are used in and their importance, it is time to list down the Essential oils and the corresponding complications they are used in treating for your better understanding and access.

The list below will cover the most common and the most important conditions and the corresponding Essential oils that are used to treat those conditions. This is a certified and approved list. And we have compiled it solely for your convenience.

Sr. No.	Health Complication	Essential oil/s
1	Anti-Cancer	i. Lemongrass Essential oil ii. Thyme Essential oil
2	Anti-Inflammatory	i. Lavender Essential oil
3	Anti-Oxidant	ii. Myrrh Essential oil iii. Frankincense Essential oil
4	Anti-Viral	i. Lemon Essential oil ii. Oregano Essential oil iii. Thieves Essential oil
5	Arthritis	i. Black Pepper Essential oil ii. Helichrysum Essential oil iii. Roman Chamomile Essential oil
6	Bruises	i. Helichrysum Essential oil
7	Cold and Fever	i. Bay Laurel Essential oil ii. Eucalyptus Essential oil iii. Lavender Essential oil iv. Peppermint Essential oil v. Ravensara Essential oil
8	Cough	i. Bay Laurel Essential oil ii. Eucalyptus Essential oil iii. Lavender Essential oil iv. Peppermint Essential oil v. Ravensara Essential oil vi. Thieves Essential oil
9	Crohn's Disease	i. Basil Essential oil ii. Peppermint Essential oil
10	Headache	i. Lavender Essential oil ii. Marjoram Essential oil iii. Peppermint Essential oil iv. Roman Chamomile Essential oil
11	Hormone Regulation	i. Thyme Essential oil
12	Influenza	i. Oregano Essential oil ii. Thieves Essential oil

13	Lyme Disease	i.	Cinnamon Essential oil
		ii.	Clove Essential oil
		iii.	Frankincense Essential oil
		iv.	Garlic Essential oil
		v.	Geranium Essential oil
		vi.	Lavender Essential oil
		vii.	Marjoram Essential oil
		viii.	Oregano Essential oil
		ix.	Rose Essential oil
		x.	Rosemary Essential oil
		xi.	Tea Tree Essential oil
		xii.	Thyme Essential oil
		xiii.	Vetiver Essential oil
14	Menstrual Cramps	i.	Cypress Essential oil
		ii.	Lavender Essential oil
		iii.	Peppermint Essential oil
15	Nausea	i.	Peppermint Essential oil
		ii.	Spearmint Essential oil
16	Sore muscles	i.	Black Pepper Essential oil
		ii.	Clary Sage Essential oil
		iii.	German Chamomile Essential oil
		iv.	Ginger Essential oil
		v.	Helichrysum Essential oil
17	Sleep	i.	Lavender Essential oil
		ii.	Jasmine Essential oil
		iii.	Marjoram Essential oil
		iv.	Neroli Essential oil
		v.	Roman Chamomile Essential oil
18	Stuffy Nose	i.	Eucalyptus Essential oil
		ii.	Peppermint Essential oil
		iii.	Ravensara Essential oil

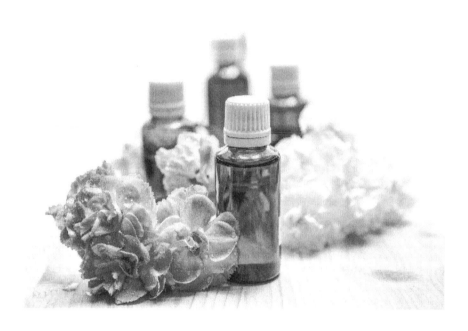

CHAPTER 7

AROMATIC COMPOSITIONS

So, you have read past chapter 5 and 6. Wohoo!

In the chapter, No. 7 Aromatic Compositions, we are going to learn about the recipes of performing aromatherapy. Yes, you heard it right. You will learn to cook. Kidding!

You will learn to prepare the Aromatherapy mix. We will discuss a few everyday use Aromatherapy mix recipes. The purpose of it is to enable you to perform aromatherapy with ease at home, and we will provide you the right directions, compositions, and instructions.

Sounds cool? It is.

1. Aromatherapy Recipe for treating Arthritis
2. Aromatherapy Recipe for treating Bruises
3. Aromatherapy Recipe for treating Congestion and Sinuses or Stuffy Nose
4. Aromatherapy Recipe for treating Menstrual Cramps
5. Aromatherapy Recipe for Cough, Cold and Flu
6. Aromatherapy Recipe for Treating Acne
7. Aromatherapy Recipe for Facial toner
8. Aromatherapy Recipe for treating Scrapes
9. Aromatherapy Recipe for Treating Insomnia
10. Aromatherapy Recipe for Treating Depression
11. Aromatherapy Recipe for Treating Anxiety

Aromatherapy Recipes for Various Health Complications

Aromatherapy is a science in itself. A lot of research and investment is required to get the right information and perform the right techniques. Here are a few common health conditions that need attention discussed below. The recipes are tried, tested and verified. Learn, Enjoy and Perform Aromatherapy at home.

1. Arthritis

For treating Arthritis, we can prepare two different blends. Both the blends can be used alone or mixed together depending upon the choice of the user.

Blend No. 1

Blend No. 1 will contain the following ingredients in the corresponding quantities written along with them.

  i.   Black Pepper Essential oil – 4 drops
 ii.   Roman Chamomile Essential oil – 20 drops
iii.   Carrier oil – 2 fluid ounces

Blend No. 2

Blend No. 2 will contain the following ingredients in the corresponding quantities written along with them.

  i.   Helichrysum Essential oil – 10 drops
 ii.   Roman Chamomile Essential oil – 10 drops
iii.   Carrier oil – 2 fluid ounces

Usage Directions

A small quantity of either Blend No. 1 or Blend No. 2 or both mixed together is used to massage around the arthritic joints. The massage techniques should be discussed with the aromatherapy practitioner prior application to avoid any discomfort and pain.

Choice of a Carrier oil

Following Carrier oils can be the choice for arthritic pain,

  a. Hemp seed oil
  b. Jojoba oil

c. Pomegranate oil

In addition to these, a vegetable oil (not a carrier oil) called the emu oil can be used because of its anti-inflammatory properties.

2. Bruises

For treating the bruises and prevention of scar formation, the following aromatherapy blend is to be used.

Aromatherapy Blend

Aromatherapy blend for treating bruises will contain the following ingredients in the corresponding quantities written along with them.

    i.   Helichrysum Essential oil – 8 drops
    ii.   Carrier oil – 1 fluid ounce

Usage Directions

Create the blend and store it in a dark colored bottle. Apply the blend lightly on the bruises 1 to 2 times a day.

Choice of a Carrier oil

The following carrier oils can be used for treating bruises

    a. Jojoba oil
    b. Sweet Almond oil

3. Congestion and Sinuses (Stuffy Nose)

For treating stuffy nose, a three essential oil aromatherapy blend is used that can either be used via Aromatherapy diffuser, inhaler or via cotton ball. It will relieve a person from congestion and sinuses.

Aromatherapy Blend

Aromatherapy blend for treating stuffy nose will contain the following ingredients in the corresponding quantities written along with them.

  i.   Eucalyptus Essential oil – 30 drops
  ii. Peppermint Essential oil – 4 drops
  iii. Ravensara Essential oil – 26 drops

Usage Directions

The blend is produced and stored in a dark colored bottle. The blend is then either used via aromatherapy diffuser; the blend is diffused and inhaled. It can in other way be used via soaking a cotton ball with the blend and placed near the nostrils. The blend is then inhaled and will relieve the stuffy nose.

Choice of Carrier oil

No carrier oil is required for the treatment of stuffy nose or congestion and sinuses.

4. Menstrual Cramps

The period suffering, menstrual pain, menstrual cramps are not a new thing. Almost every woman go through it once a month in her life starting from puberty till menopause.

Aromatherapy Blend

Aromatherapy blend for treating menstrual pain will contain the following ingredients in the corresponding quantities written along with them.

    i.   Cypress Essential oil – 4 drops
    ii.   Lavender Essential oil – 3 drops
    iii. Peppermint Essential oil – 5 drops
    iv. Carrier oil – 1 fluid ounce

Usage Directions

Mix all the ingredients well making a blend, and then store it in a dark colored bottle for protection. When needed, that is, during menstruation and cramps, take a small amount of this blend and gently massage it on to the affected part that is hurting. This part mostly is the abdominal area.

Choice of a Carrier oil

For the treatment and relief of menstrual cramps, the following carrier oil can be a choice

    a. Jojoba oil

5. Cough, Cold and Flu

For treating cough, cold and flu; a similar blend can be used. The aromatherapy recipe is composed of a minimum of four to seven essential oils. The aromatherapy blend we will be discussing below will contain four essential oils. It is used via Aromatherapy diffuser, diffused in the atmosphere and inhaled killing the germs outside as well as inside. It will relieve a person from cough, cold and flu.

Aromatherapy Blend

Aromatherapy blend for treating cough, cold and flu will contain the following ingredients in the corresponding quantities written along with them.

   i.   Bay Laurel Essential oil – 2 drops
   ii. Eucalyptus Essential oil – 5 drops
   iii. Lavender Essential oil – 5 drops
   iv. Ravensara Essential oil – 3 drops

Usage Direction

The blend is produced and stored in a dark colored bottle. The blend is then either used via aromatherapy diffuser; the blend is diffused and inhaled. This blend is supposed to be diffused in the area throughout the season of cough, cold and flu.

Choice of a Carrier oil

No carrier oil is required in the preventive measure and for the treatment of cough, cold and flu.

6. Acne

For treating the acne and prevention of scar formation, an exquisite aromatherapy blend with proper research is required. The following aromatherapy blend is to be used for this purpose.

Aromatherapy Blend

Aromatherapy blend for treating acne will contain the following ingredients in the corresponding quantities written along with them.

  i.   Lavender Essential oil – 6 drops
  ii. Tea Tree Essential oil – 5 drops
  iii. Geranium Essential oil – 1 drop
  iv. Carrier oil – 1 fluid ounce

Usage Directions

Create the blend and store it in a dark colored bottle with a dropper top. Before use, roll it for 2 minutes to mix the blend perfectly. Apply the blend lightly on the acne or acne-prone areas avoiding ear, eyes, nose, and nostrils. Apply 1 to 2 times a day depending upon the need. For best results, use it with aromatherapy facial toner.

Choice of a Carrier oil

The following carrier oils can be used for treating acne.

  a. Jojoba oil
  b. Fractionated Coconut oil

7. Recipe for Facial toner

A facial toner is a necessity when it comes to treating the acne and prevention of scar formation. However, what would be better than a natural aromatherapy toner. An exquisite aromatherapy blend with proper research is required. The following aromatherapy blend is to be used for this purpose.

Aromatherapy Blend

Aromatherapy blend for facial toner will contain the following ingredients in the corresponding quantities written along with them.

i. Grapefruit Essential oil – 8 drops
ii. Tea Tree Essential oil – 4 drops
iii. Cypress Essential oil – 4 drops
iv. Hydrosol – 2.5 fluid ounce
v. High Proof Vodka – 1 fluid ounce

Usage Directions

Create the blend in a 4 oz. bottle, adding everything in it. Mix it well. A 3.5 fl. oz. of toner will be produced while the rest of the space will let you mix the blend well. Apply the toner on the face or other acne-prone areas avoiding eyes. Apply 1 to 2 times a day depending upon the need.

Choice of a Hydrosol

The following hydrosol is required for creating an aromatherapy facial toner for treating acne.

a. Witch Hazel Hydrosol

8. Scrapes and Cuts

For treating the cuts and scrapes while keeping the prevention of scar formation in mind, a complete and exquisite aromatherapy balm is required. The following aromatherapy blend is to be used for this purpose.

Aromatherapy Balm

Aromatherapy balm for treating scrapes and cuts will contain the following ingredients in the corresponding quantities written along with them.

i.   Lavender Essential oil – 40 drops
ii. Tea Tree Essential oil – 40 drops
iii. Grated Beeswax – 1 net. wt. ounce
iv. Wide-mouthed jar – 4 ounces
v.   Carrier oil – 3 fluid ounces

Usage Directions

Melt the beeswax in double boiler. When it is done, add in the heated carrier and infused oils and stir until mixed well. When done with it, add in lavender and tea tree essential oils, and mix it well.

When the stirring is done, add in the jar and let it cool. Add in lid afterwards. Make sure the balm is cool before using it. Apply the balm lightly on the scrapes and cuts and apply bandage depending upon the need.

Choice of a Carrier oil or Infused oil

The following carrier oils can be used for treating cuts and scrapes.

    a. Jojoba oil
    b. Sweet Almond oil
    c. Calendula oil

9. For Relieving Anxiety

Anxiety is killing the generation along with depression and insomnia. These three calls for an immediate therapy and cure to save individuals. For relieving anxiety, the aromatherapy blend should provide the required benefits. The following aromatherapy blend is to be used for this purpose.

Aromatherapy Blend

Aromatherapy blend for relieving anxiety will contain the following ingredients in the corresponding quantities written along with them.

Blend # 1

    i.   Bergamot Essential oil – 2 drops

    ii.   Sandalwood Essential oil – 3 drops

Blend # 2

    i.   Bergamot Essential oil – 2 drops

    ii.   Clary Sage Essential oil – 2 drops

    iii. Frankincense Essential oil – 1 drop

Blend # 3

    i.   Clary Sage Essential oil – 3 drops

    ii.   Lavender Essential oil – 2 drops

Blend # 4

    i.   Rose Essential oil – 1 drop

    ii.   Lavender Essential oil – 1 drop

    iii. Mandarin Essential oil – 2 drops

    iv. Vetiver Essential oil – 1 drop

Usage Directions

Create the blend and store it in a dark colored bottle. Any of the above-mentioned blends can be used. Usage can be by any of the following methods

a) Diffuser Blend
b) Bath Oil
c) Bath Salts
d) Massage Oil
e) Air Freshener

Choice of a Carrier oil

No carrier oil is required in the treatment of insomnia and sleeplessness.

10. Insomnia

Insomnia is killing the generation with anxiety and depression. These three calls for an immediate therapy and cure to save individuals. For treating insomnia or sleeplessness, the aromatherapy blend should provide the required benefits. The following aromatherapy blend is to be used for this purpose.

Aromatherapy Blend

Aromatherapy blend for treating insomnia will contain the following ingredients in the corresponding quantities written along with them.

i.   Bergamot Essential oil – 5 drops
ii.   Clary Sage Essential oil – 5 drops
iii. Roman Chamomile Essential oil – 10 drops

Usage Directions

Create the blend and store it in a dark colored bottle with a dropper top. Before use, roll it for 2 minutes to mix the blend perfectly. Apply the blend 2-3 drops on a tissue or cotton and place it under your pillow. This will aid in falling to sleep. Avoid direct contact with eyes and face.

A diffuser method is another good and preferred option. Add essential oils in 1:1:2 ratio or better drops respectively in your diffuser. An additional of 1-2 drops of lavender oil will aid in relaxation and drowsiness, however, more than this would trigger an opposite effect.

Choice of a Carrier oil

No carrier oil is required in the treatment of insomnia and sleeplessness.

11. Depression

Depression is killing the generation with anxiety and insomnia. These three calls for an immediate therapy and cure to save individuals. For treating depression, the aromatherapy blend should provide the required benefits. The following aromatherapy blend is to be used for this purpose.

Aromatherapy Blend

Aromatherapy blend for treating depression will contain the following ingredients in the corresponding quantities written along with them.

Blend # 1

   i.   Orange Essential oil – 1 drop
   ii.   Rose Essential oil – 1 drop
   iii. Sandalwood Essential oil – 3 drops

Blend # 2

   i.   Bergamot Essential oil – 3 drops
   ii.   Clary Sage Essential oil – 2 drops

Blend # 3

   i.   Grapefruit Essential oil – 3 drops
   ii.   Lavender Essential oil – 1 drop
   iii. Ylang Ylang Essential oil – 1 drop

Blend # 4

i.   Frankincense Essential oil – 2 drops
ii. Lemon Essential oil – 1 drop
iii. Jasmine Essential oil – 2 drops
iv. Neroli Essential oil – 2 drops

Usage Directions

Create the blend and store it in a dark colored bottle. Any of the above-mentioned blends can be used. Usage can be by any of the following methods

a) Diffuser Blend
b) Bath Oil
c) Bath Salts
d) Massage Oil
e) Air Freshener

Choice of a Carrier oil

No carrier oil is required in the treatment of insomnia and sleeplessness.

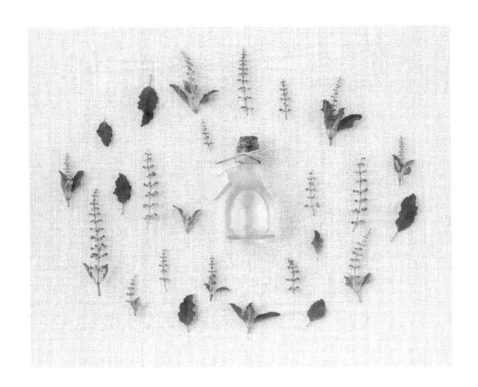

CONCLUSION

Hast, it just Ended? Oh Yeah! You came this far, Congratulations! We made it.

Now, you have learned almost all about Essential oils. Starting from the Introduction to Aromatherapy, Essential oils to their Aromatic Ingredients, Aromatic Compositions, safe levels, and Recipes. You Know Everything Now!

We told you in the Beginning that You will get the Ultimate guide to cherish the rest of your life and will never regret it. We meant it!

This made you understand not only the itty-bitty details about the ingredients, procedures but also the Recipes. Can we talk about them? Now you are able to deal with illnesses like Arthritis, Bruises, Congestion, and Stuffy Nose, Menstrual Cramps, Cough, Cold and Flu, Acne, Scrapes, and Cuts.

Not only this, you can make your best facial toner at home as well. To add cherry on top, your long pained and untreatable Insomnia, Depression, and Anxiety can now stay away from you. You have found the right path.

We are so glad we made it together till the end, and we are so grateful you trusted us. We are equally excited for you to kill the taboo; fight these conditions and live the best life You Deserve!

In the end, (too soon) we would like to thank you and wish you all the best for your health and happiness. And Remember,

"Essential oils and Aromatherapy can do for you that nothing else can because Nature has power."

You deserve way more than this. Stay Happy, Stay Healthy, and Enjoy Life to its Fullest. Nobody isn't going to get it again, Right?

Know Your Worth!

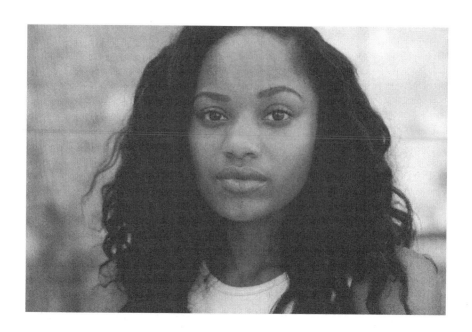

ABOUT THE AUTHOR

AMANDA ROBINSON is an experienced coach, trainer, a life-style blogger, freelance writer, and books author.

Amanda is passionate about fun, simple, healthy living and knows tons of tips and tricks about decluttering, money saving, life style improving.

Amanda lives in California with her husband and three children. While not spending time with kids, inventing new life hacks and writing new books, Amanda loves practicing jogging, photographing and exploring local farmer's market.

Find other my books on Amazon!

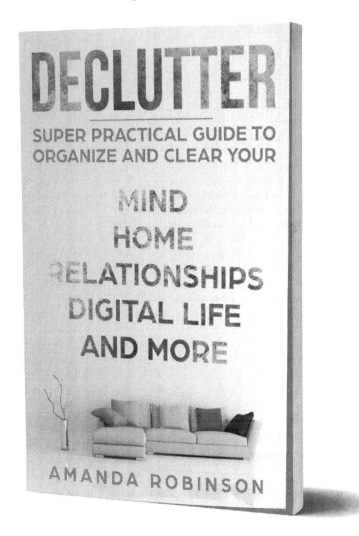

Please leave feedback if you love them!
It is very important for me

Printed in Great Britain
by Amazon